# PLAN NOW
# & SAVE YOUR
# ASS(ETS) LATER!

ALEX KINCAID, J.D.

www.AlexKincaidLaw.com

*Praise for*
**Plan Now & Save Your Ass(ets) Later!**

"An entertaining and educational book written by an attorney who has devoted her life to helping others." – *A. Tompkins*

"This book finally got my mom and dad to plan! Worth every penny!" – T. *Bailey*

"Everyone who is questioning which route to take for estate planning needs to read this book. It gave me direction and prepared me for the estate planning process." – *S. Michaelson*

"I shared this with my grandfather, and he created his plan in two months. It helped guide him in the right direction, gave him confidence, and gave us all peace of mind." – *A. Rodriguez*

"This book made me realize I have had the wrong estate plan for my family. With Alex's help, I was able to find a plan that was perfect for my family and made sure my ex-son-in-law won't get rich." ☺ – *M. Anderson*

"Finally! A comprehensible book that helps!" – *S.L.*

"Great read, provided lots of information, and answered questions I didn't know I had!" – *J. Toluse*

## DISCLAIMER

Please keep in mind that reading a book is not a substitute for legal advice. As this book portrays, the laws pertaining to estate planning are vast, and this book only provides generalities about common estate planning issues. This book is only a guide, designed to provide general information regarding trusts and estates.

The author, publisher, and copyright owner expressly disclaim any liability for errors or omissions that may be in this book and assume no responsibility for any harm that comes from the use or application of information in this book. The laws pertaining to trusts and estates are constantly evolving, and there are many technical and gray areas to all laws. While I have made an effort to have the information in this book up to date at the time of publication, you must remember that laws change—you cannot simply rely on what is written in this book as the law. The reader should instead rely on professional advice before proceeding with any legal decisions. As the author, even though I am an attorney, I am not providing legal advice or other legal services. Just because you are reading this book does not mean you are my client. Guidance on how to hire me or my firm can be found on my website: www.AlexKincaidLaw.com.

The case studies revealed in this book have been changed as necessary to protect client confidentiality.

The best plans rely upon having the best people to discuss and carry out the plans. This book is dedicated to my husband, Eric, because he is my best friend, and the one I rely on each and every day with little plans and big plans. It is also dedicated to my sister, Alison, because we are constantly planning, and to Jenni Forsyth, who is planning to make history. I am blessed to have you in my life.

## ACKNOWLEDGEMENTS

Thank you to Jenni Forsyth, Christel Schumacher, Wendy Breckon, and Joe Toluse.

# Table of Contents

# 1
# A FAILURE TO PLAN IS
# A PLAN TO FAIL

Over the course of my 20 year legal career, I learned lessons in estate planning from different sources. These sources included my own clients and cases, educational classes I attended, discussions with my elder law colleagues, and reading a wide variety of books and treatises.

Ironically, I drew some of the most valuable information about estate planning from the cases I prosecuted during my early years as a criminal law attorney. Why would I gain estate planning knowledge from criminal cases? Because far too many criminals make a living by scamming the elderly.

Over 60% of the population in the county where I served as the elected District Attorney consisted of senior citizens. In the courthouse of this retirement community, my eyes were opened to a group of crime victims that many people never suspect: senior citizens. Seniors can be especially vulnerable to criminals, because they are an easy target for criminals who are quick to recognize when a senior citizen has anything worth stealing, is easily manipulated, trusting, and lonely.

These criminals are not always strangers. I witnessed neighbors, caretakers, and family members become cold and vicious when money was available.

I also saw the failure of the government-controlled court system to protect many seniors, simply because by the time the court was involved, it was too late to protect them from the criminals who had already struck. In the cases I reviewed and prosecuted, the money was already gone, and the mentally incapacitated victims were frequently unable to testify about what had happened. Some of the victims could not remember the particulars of why they gave someone money. Sometimes, they had no recollection of giving money away at all. Some of these cases went unprosecuted, because without a victim who could testify, there simply was no case that could be proven to a jury.

In almost every one of these instances, proper planning on the part of the senior could have prevented the abuse. For these seniors, lack of planning opened the door for a multitude of complications, including theft, fraud, and physical abuse. Elder abuse can often be prevented with a competent estate plan in place, where a trusted person can step in and protect the senior before the crime occurs.

The following two cases show how the failure to plan allowed two criminals to make money from the unsuspecting senior citizens.

**The Nigerian Nabber.** One day at my office, I received a phone call from a frantic woman in California, who claimed her mom's bank had just called her to warn her that her mom had wired the money in her small savings account ($35,000.00) to a man in Nigeria. The bank was not able to stop the Western Union transaction. They had no information that their customer was unable to make her own decisions, although they clearly knew she was being scammed. The victim (the caller's mother) had no estate plan. She had no agent under a power of attorney, a trustee who could step in and take charge of her assets, or anyone else who was named to be in a position to protect her. This 80-year-old woman's life's savings was suddenly 100% gone. All the daughter could do in response to the bank's call was go to court after the tragedy had struck and ask the judge to put her in charge of her mom's remaining assets, which consisted of her small home, a car, and her monthly social security check.

**"Concerned" Neighbors.** The neighbor and friend of an elderly multi-millionaire, who lived in an ocean-view condominium complex, became concerned when he found out his friend had been giving away large sums of cash to people knocking on his door.

These criminals knocked on their victim's door to "remind" him that they had bought groceries or paid a bill for him. They told this unsuspecting, wealthy man with dementia that he had promised to pay them back for their help. This elderly gentleman was embarrassed at his failure to repay such kind people, and when they stood at his door, would retrieve some cash from his house "cash stash" immediately and hand it to them.

One day, when a knock came on his door, his true friend was sitting in the living room and overheard one of these exchanges. After multiple phone calls to senior services, law enforcement, attorneys, and the man's own two sons, no one wanted to take on the role as the senior citizen's court-appointed conservator, who would be in a position to control his money and protect him from further crimes. This senior had no estate plan in place. He had failed to plan, and criminals were taking advantage of him on a daily basis. He had left his own protection to the government-controlled court system, which struggled to find a solution to protect him. Finally, the friend who reported the ordeal to law enforcement agreed to act as his conservator. The appointment was, in some ways, too late, because the senior had already been repeatedly victimized.

# 2
# DON'T RELY ON THE COURT SYSTEM (PROBATE)

Like the senior citizens I described in the first chapter, you may not have a plan. If that is the case, the government has a plan for you. The government's plan is called "probate." Every state in the country has a "probate code," which is a set of laws that dictates whom a judge must put in charge to manage your assets and make medical decisions for you if you are incapacitated, and who will manage your estate and inherit your assets when you die. This probate system is the government's default way of dealing with people who do not plan for themselves.

Too many people believe that the court exists to protect them. The reality is that the courts are a place of last resort for people who have no other option. Let's face it: Courts are clogged, inefficient "justice" systems where most people who experience a court process do not feel they received justice at all.

The government-controlled court system exists to allow victims to come forward and *attempt* to recover some of their losses. The courts cannot and do not prevent the tragedies. Sometimes, the courts cannot even prevent situations they know are happening.

For example, I was once contacted by a family member who had consulted with a paralegal (not a licensed attorney) to obtain guardianship of her mother. The paralegal's paperwork did not supply the court with the required information under state law, so even though this person's mother was in the hospital after lying in her own bed, unattended, for so long that she had maggots in her back, the court refused to approve the guardianship.

This case is a prime example of why I decided to help people plan their affairs. After serving as a trial attorney for almost a decade, it was clear to me that the courthouse is a place of tragedy – people seldom achieve justice in court. The best that most people who resort to the court can hope for is to achieve some kind of settlement or retribution from the wrongdoer; but, most of the time, they will only realize an unsatisfactory pay-out after paying thousands of dollars in attorney fees. The old saying that an ounce of planning is worth a pound of cure holds true, especially when the planning will help you avoid this broken system.

Let us discuss what "probate" means. Probate courts oversee two main types of cases. First, a person may become incapacitated and require the court to appoint someone who can make legal decisions for the incapacitated person (a "living" probate). Second, when a person dies, the court will oversee the distribution of the dead person's (the decedent's) property.

First, let us discuss incapacity and the living probate. Statistically, at age 30, you are almost twice as likely to become injured or incapacitated as you are to die. This risk of incapacity grows with age – nearly doubling by the time you reach the age of 50. But when most people think about an estate plan, they think that the main purpose of preparing a plan is to pass their property to their family, friends, or charities after they die. While passing an inheritance is certainly a worthy consideration, an equally worthy consideration is to prepare a plan for your incapacity, which can help you avoid becoming a victim.

When people owns assets (such as a car, a home, or bank account) in their own names and become unable to manage financial affairs due to mental or physical incapacity, only a court appointee can sign or otherwise make binding decisions for the disabled person. This is true even if the person has a will, because a will can only go into effect after death. With some assets, especially real estate, all owners must sign to sell or refinance the property. So, for example, if a married couple owns their assets jointly, and one of them becomes disabled when an asset needs to be sold or refinanced, the spouse that is not disabled will have to go through the probate court in order to be granted the power to act on behalf of his or her disabled spouse.

This court process is called a living probate, because while it is similar to the probate process at death, the person who needs the court's protection is still alive. Living probates can be costly, time consuming, and cumbersome, with annual accountings, bonds, reports, ongoing determinations of incapacity and incompetency, and fees for attorneys, accountants, doctors, and guardians. All costs are paid from the disabled person's assets, and all assets and proceedings become part of the court's (often public) probate record. A living probate usually lasts until the person recovers or dies, which, depending on his or her age when the disability begins, can be years.

The living probate process usually plays out like this: If you can no longer care for yourself, once someone notices that something is wrong, that person will need to petition (ask in writing in a specific format) the court to request that the court name someone who can make healthcare and financial decisions for you. Most states refer to this court-appointed person as the guardian and conservator, respectively.

A guardian is a person who makes day to day living decisions for you (including whether you will stay in your own home or be moved into an assisted living facility or a nursing home). A conservator is in charge of your finances and assets. In order for a person to be appointed as your guardian and conservator, they have to be willing to take on those roles, and someone has to prove in court that you are no longer able to make your own decisions or care for yourself. If you are mentally incompetent, you do not have much say over who will be appointed, because the judge does not believe you are able to make your own decisions. Instead, the judge will look at the information that is provided in the paperwork requesting the appointment of a guardian and conservator, and will make a decision.

If more than one person is asking to be appointed, or if someone objects to the appointment of a person who is asking to be appointed, the court will hold a hearing, where the interested people can present evidence, testify, and argue their positions to the judge. The person asking that you no longer be allowed to manage your own affairs can be anyone: a neighbor, a friend, a caretaker, or even an estranged child.

If you have not planned, you do not know if the person appointed will be someone you trust, knows your wishes, or has good judgment. The judge may never hear the information that you know. You have the opportunity before you ever become reliant on the assistance of others to make these decisions to put your wishes in writing. The process of making these decisions final before anything happens is part of creating an estate plan.

Estate planning allows you to keep control, even if you are incapacitated, because 1) you either tell the court who you would like to manage your affairs if you are ever not able to care for yourself, or, 2) if you create a trust (more on this later), you will completely remove the court from the process and create a binding, legal document designating your choices. In your estate planning documents, you will spell out what it means to be incapacitated, and even who should make the decision that you can no longer care for yourself. Should it be your spouse, a spouse and a doctor, a spouse and a child, two doctors? You have the ability to name your trusted people ahead of time. Your named people will take the place of the judge.

A similar path is followed by the probate court after you die. Someone will need to file a request with the court to be in charge of your assets (think of assets as anything you own when you died – your home, your car, your firearms, your pets). The court will look at the probate laws in your state to decide whom the judge must put in charge of your assets, and where your assets should ultimately go. These laws do not take into consideration whether or not you have a relationship with all of your children, or whether a child has a particular problem, such as drug addiction.

In other words, probate means that when you die, a court will impose default laws that do not take your specific situation into consideration. This usually means that all biological or legally adopted children will be treated equally (including the gambler, drug addict, or child you never met or who has lost contact with you, while step-children are ignored). Any pet animals are treated as mere personal property by the probate laws– no different than a car or other object, and they may or may not have a dollar-value that makes them important to anyone involved in the probate proceeding.

Simple, "quick" probates usually last six months to a year before they are completed, and probates cost at least a couple of thousand dollars or much more, depending on where you live. More complicated probates can last three to five years (or more). I was once involved in a probate that included 15 different lawyers, each representing a different heir. My attorney fees alone for representing the personal representative (also known as an "executor" or "executrix") and defending what the testator (the author of a will) wrote in his "simple will" came to over $150,000.00. The money to pay these fees came from the estate. If these fees seem high, consider that a judge awarded these fees to my firm as completely reasonable in light of all the fighting between the heirs. This case took place over a decade ago.

To get the court to help you or your loved ones, whether you are incapacitated or you die, your loved ones will need to understand many rules. These rules include requirements for any paperwork filed with the court, what evidence can be presented, what must be proven in court, when and how to file the paperwork, whom to give copies of the paperwork, and when to show up for a hearing in front of the judge.

Most people have to hire an attorney to explain the rules to them and guide them through the court process. Attorneys are expensive. Many people cannot afford an attorney. Some people go in debt to hire an attorney to fight their case, only to wind up settling when the case takes too long, is too stressful, or is too expensive to complete. Settling a case frequently happens after someone has started a lawsuit, and months or years go by without any "justice" ever being accomplished. The court is simply another government-controlled, broken system. It is, again, a place of last resort.

Why would you want to use a government system when you can create your own system, with your own rules?  Many people never realize they have this option.

Even worse, many people do not realize all the ways they can wind up in probate court, which include:

1) They do not plan at all;

2) They only create a last will and testament;

3) They rely on a durable power of attorney for their incapacity plan (especially if the durable power of attorney is generic and short);

4) Their plan fails for any reason, such as not naming an alternate person to be in charge, not signing certain documents in front of a notary or witnesses, or kids who argue that they did not know what they were doing when they signed their estate planning documents.

Lawyers who were fed up with the inefficiencies of the court system created the living trust to protect their clients and their clients' assets from the inefficient, public, court probate system.

# 3
# WILLS VS. TRUSTS

People often call my office and tell my receptionist that they would like to prepare a will. I have realized over the years that most people do not fully understand what will happen after they die if they rely on a will to carry out their wishes. They also have little, if any, understanding of all the options they have before them. They are simply thinking that they would like to put something in writing about what they would like to happen after their death.

There are many options for putting your wishes in writing. The most basic question everyone must answer is whether to create a will-based plan or a trust-based plan.

Trust planning is a type of estate plan where you can complete all the hard work now, but the process is simplified for your loved ones later. Will planning is less work for you now, but the process is usually more complicated (and expensive) later. Trusts cost more to set up, but you avoid the costs associated with the court system later. For clients who have family members who will disagree, or whose powers of attorney are not sufficient, the costs of a well-written living trust plan are far less than the costs of writing a will-based plan that winds up in probate. For others, the cost may be similar, and the difference is simply whether you pay now or pay later. In other words, will planning versus trust planning means paying more to set up the trust and do the hard work now, or paying less to set up a simple will but paying for the probate of that will later.

What are the other differences between wills and trusts? Think of a will as a letter to the judge. Instead of relying on the state default system and its rules, you are writing to the judge to let the judge know whom you would like to be in charge of your affairs when you are gone, and who should receive any assets you leave behind. A will essentially states, "Dear Judge, When I die, please do the following."

For a judge to consider what you write in this letter, there must be some proof that you wrote it. The state's laws where you signed your will determine whether or not there is enough proof. Most states require that a will be witnessed by at least two people, and that those witnesses swear that you were of legal age, sound mind (you understood what you were signing, who your family members are, and what your assets are), and that you were not being forced to sign the will (under coercion or duress). Those witnesses must swear to these facts before a notary.

You may be able to write a will in your own handwriting, but the acceptance of such "holographic" wills is rare. Even if a court accepts a handwritten will, handwritten wills more easily come under attack, because they usually do not have the sworn statements of witnesses who can testify that you willingly and knowingly wrote the will. These wills are, in a word, "suspect."

After you die, your will is filed with the court, and property that is in your name without a beneficiary designation (like a bank account) will be transferred according to what you wrote in your will. The probate process varies depending on where the probate is filed, because each state has a different set of probate laws.

Even though the specific rules may differ from state to state, some generalities about probate hold true across the country. Probates are usually filed where you died, where you resided, or where you owned property. A will also does not provide any kind of incapacity plan. If you are ever unable to manage your own affairs, because you can no longer make your own decisions or are physically unable to take care of yourself, the will does nothing to help you.

If you create a will, you will need additional planning for your potential incapacity, or you may wind up in the court system for a living probate, with a judge appointing a guardian or a conservator to make decisions for you. The most common incapacity planning documents that are created along with a will are a health care power of attorney and living will and a durable power of attorney. These documents are each discussed in more detail in a later chapter. While these documents can help avoid a living probate, they often do not, as is explained later.

Most of my clients would prefer to confidently wipe the entire court process out of the picture, which is why I am usually preparing a living trust as the cornerstone of a client's estate plan. Think of a trust as your opportunity to write your own rulebook. The rulebook is a plan for your incapacity and for what will happen when you die. When you create this rulebook, you are completely replacing the government-controlled court system, where a judge will oversee your affairs if you are incapacitated and oversee the court process that will take place when you die. These are the guardianship and conservatorship and estate proceedings mentioned above that will take place in the clogged, inefficient, public, and expensive "probate" court.

Instead of state default laws dictating who will be in charge and where your assets will go, your trust will tell people who is in charge if you are incapacitated, how you should be taken care of, and who will be in charge and where your property will go when you die. Trusts that are correctly written and funded (meaning that your property is re-titled in the name of the trust), will completely take the place of the government-controlled court system and the probate process.

If you prepare a living trust, your incapacity plan can prevent the need for a guardianship or conservatorship. This is because a living trust will go a step beyond simply naming your preferred helpers and granting those helpers the power to act for you. The living trust goes beyond these basics by also providing detailed direction on *how* you wish to receive care. For example, most of my clients clearly state in their trust that they will remain in their own home for as long as possible, that if they need an assisted living arrangement, in-home caregivers should be hired first, and if they need to be in a new home, they name the location or even the specific place where they would like to reside. These detailed directions will avoid arguing amongst children, or spouses and children from another relationship.

A fully funded revocable living trust avoids a living probate because when a living trust is established, the titles of assets (such as the deed to your house) are changed from the current owner's individual name (you, if you create the trust) to the name of the trustee (manager) of the trust. This is called "funding" the trust. If the trust has been fully funded (all titles changed), and the person (you, if you create the trust) becomes unable to conduct business (make your own decisions), there is no reason for a living probate, because the trust creator does not own any assets in his or her name. The "successor trustee," hand-picked by you when you wrote the trust to manage your assets, can automatically step in, without court interference, and manage your financial affairs—sell or refinance assets to help pay for long-term care, keep your business running, manage the family farm, do whatever needs to be done, for as long as needed. All of this takes place without anyone having to go to court.

With a trust, you can plan for your loved ones. You can plan for your pets. You can put everything that is important to you in writing, on paper, to make sure that your wishes are carried out. That is what estate planning is all about.

When I explain the difference between relying upon a last will and testament coupled with a general durable power of attorney versus relying upon a revocable living trust to my clients, I focus on the power the client is taking back from the government: You create the rules with your trust, not the government. A trust completely bypasses the court system. Trust planning is a legal way of taking control of your own affairs and possessions if you die or become incapacitated.

Let us contrast the steps that take place with a trust if you are incapacitated with the steps we followed for a living probate in the last chapter. Your trust alone spells out what "incapacity" means, who decides whether you are ever incapacitated, and who steps in to manage the trust property and provide assistance to you if you become incapacitated. You can also provide detailed instructions directing your named successor trustee (think of this person as the person who will manage the trust assets for you if you cannot) on what to do with the trust assets upon your incapacity. If you become incapacitated, rather than entrusting a judge with the power over deciding who will be appointed as your guardian or conservator, what kind of care you should receive, how your assets will be dealt with, and hoping the judge does the right thing, you dictate all of these terms when you create a trust.

In other words, when you create a trust plan, your trusted people decide if you are ever incapacitated in accordance with a definition that you write in your trust. If those people agree that you can no longer manage your own affairs (in other words, take care of yourself by remembering to take medication or to pay your bills on time, for example), they sign paperwork indicating this and will now have control of your assets to protect you. All of this happens without the court system involved.

A similar situation occurs when you die. Instead of the court ordering who is in charge and where your assets will go, your trusted person, whom you named in your trust as your successor trustee, will sign a document accepting his or her role and responsibility as your successor trustee. That notarized document takes the place of a court order appointing a personal representative (also known as an executor or executrix). The goal with trust planning is usually to completely remove the court system from your affairs if you are incapacitated or die.

In summary, if you become incapacitated, you do not have to leave your personal affairs to the courts to figure out through a time-consuming process involving the public airing of your affairs. The same is true upon death. Why leave a last will and testament that allows a judge you do not know to oversee what happens to your assets, when you can create your own system via a trust instead? With a properly constructed trust plan, you have created your own plan for incapacity and death, and the people you choose can step in and follow your plan when something happens to you.

As we discuss in later chapters, there are many kinds of trusts. The most common (and basic) kind of trust is called a revocable living trust. This kind of trust was designed by attorneys in an effort to avoid the probate process after death. These trusts are specifically designed to take the place of a will and the court system.

# 4

# WHO SHOULD CREATE A TRUST?

For too long, Americans have been taught to rely on the government for their needs: Social security will pay your retirement. The Affordable Care Act will take care of your medical expenses. The court will handle your affairs if you are incapacitated or when you die.

As I explained in the prior chapters, the government-controlled court system is not the answer to legal problems any more than social security is the answer for living expenses during retirement. When I explain the difference between planning with a will and the planning and protection that can be done with a trust, clients almost always choose to prepare a trust, because the benefits clearly outweigh the costs.

Trusts are excellent investments for you and your family.

There is a lot of misinformation on the internet about trusts. While having an estate with a certain dollar value may be the marker for whether a client needs tax planning, it is not the marker on whether or not a client should consider a living trust. There is no dollar value that needs to be achieved to want to avoid a public, complicated, inefficient process during your or your family's most difficult times. Too many Americans are using the court system as their estate plan simply because they do not know that they have other options. One of the best options is to take control of your own affairs and plan to protect yourself, your loved ones, and your legacy with a legal document called a trust.

Instead of looking for a particular dollar value in an estate, when I meet with clients to discuss how they would like to plan their estate, I look for "red flags," which alert me to whether they would greatly benefit from a trust-based plan. These red flags often have more to do with family dynamics rather than how valuable their assets may be.

Other times, while a trust-based plan may not be necessary, it would provide the clients with peace of mind, privacy, and a streamlined system.

If any of the following apply to you, you should consider whether the benefits of a trust-based plan are for you:

1. If you have a blended family and would like to minimize problems between your spouse, your children, and your step-children;

2. If you have trouble with one or more family members and wish to ensure the problem relative is

not involved in your affairs;

3.  If you will be disinheriting a child;

4.  If you would prefer to protect a child's inheritance from creditors and predators, including divorcing spouses;

5.  If you would like to motivate a child to attend college or otherwise become a productive member of society;

6.  If you have real property in more than one state;

7.  If you have a child with special needs;

8. If you want control of the process that will take place if you become incapacitated (disabled) or die;

9.  If you prefer a private, simple process rather than a complicated, public, court process; or

10.  If you prefer to save your loved ones time, expense, and stress should anything happen to you.

Any one of the above reasons is reason enough to consider preparing a living trust.

Trust planning is about control. If you would like to avoid the government's plan for you and your family in the case that you are disabled or pass away, and you would like a streamlined, efficient process where you maximize control of what will happen and who is in charge of carrying out your wishes, then a trust should be a part of your estate plan.

# 5

# UNDERSTANDING TRUST TERMINOLOGY

A trust is a legal entity (similar to a corporation or limited liability company) created by a "grantor" for the benefit of designated "beneficiaries" and managed by at least one "trustee."

Let us take a look at these three main players in a trust.

1. **Grantor:** Depending on the state's laws, this person may be called the "settlor" or the "trustor." The grantor is simply the creator of the trust— the person who sets the trust up and signs the initial trust documents.

2. **Trustee:** Think of the trustee as the "manager" of any property titled in the name of the

trust. The grantor will decide what property is initially transferred to the trust, and the trustee will then make decisions about what can be done with the trust assets. The grantor and the trustee may be the same person, which is usually the case with a revocable living trust.

3. **Beneficiary:** A trust beneficiary is the person who enjoys the benefits of the trust assets. For example, you might set up a trust for a child. You would be the grantor, and you could also be the trustee, who manages the money for the child. You might put $100,000 in the trust for the child, and then as the trustee, you will decide where the money goes, what expenses to pay, and what to do with the trust income (adhering to any direction written in the trust). The child, however, is the beneficiary. You are only managing the trust money for the child's benefit.

There are many different kinds of trusts lawyers create for their clients, depending on what the lawyer intends to accomplish for the client. A trust may be created for tax planning, to protect young children, to save an inheritance for a disabled child, to take care of a pet, or simply to plan for the trust creator's own death and incapacity.

The most common type of estate planning trust is called a "revocable living trust." This type of trust is a plan for the person who created it (the grantor) with provisions for property management if the grantor becomes incapacitated (also called disabled) and what will happen when the grantor dies, as we discussed in detail in the last chapter.

The grantor or grantors (joint revocable living trusts are often created by spouses) transfer their assets to the trust and serve as the trustees of the trust. The grantor or trustees continue to have full control of the assets held by the trust— they can buy, sell, manage and control the trust assets just as they would if they had not transferred them to the trust. In other words, the grantor continues to conduct business as usual with respect to the assets he or she has transferred to the trust.

When the grantor dies or become incapacitated, the trust names the "successor trustee" who can step into the grantor's shoes to control the trust assets. A successor trustee can be anyone the grantor has named in the trust—a family member, friend, bank, financial advisor, or attorney. No court approval or process is required for this person to step in if the grantor dies or becomes incapacitated.

The trust will spell out who the new beneficiaries of the trust will be when the grantor dies (in other words, who inherits the trust assets). The trust assets can go directly to these beneficiaries or stay in trust for greater protection. As mentioned in other parts of this book, a properly created and funded revocable living trust will prevent the grantor from needing a court-ordered conservator if the grantor is incapacitated with respect to the trust property. The trust will also prevent the trust assets from being "probated" (having to go through the court process) when the grantor dies. This is how the creator of a revocable living trust completely removes the court from the estate plan, when set up correctly.

# 6
# NOT ALL TRUSTS ARE CREATED EQUAL

If you decide that trust planning sounds like a good option for you, your next step is to decide what kind of trust will best meet your needs. There are many different types of trusts, but an important distinction is whether a trust is revocable or irrevocable. You need to understand the differences, pros and cons, of creating a revocable living trust versus an irrevocable trust in order to make a decision about which kind (maybe both) would be best for your situation.

One day in my private law office, I met with an elderly couple who had hired an attorney to create a trust after the wife's health began declining five years earlier. This couple had a modest estate – a home, a couple of cars, a checking account, a savings account, and a monthly income they consumed each month. The wife's doctor told the couple that she would never be the same, and, in fact, her health and mental capabilities would continue to decline. The doctor was correct.

The attorney did not advise them of their options, but instead, prepared the most common type of estate planning trust – a revocable living trust. When I met with this couple five years later, the wife's condition had declined to the point that they knew she would soon need to move into a nursing home. They told me that they had already created a trust, and all of their assets were protected. They had come to see me to get advice on what steps to take next.

I reviewed their estate planning documents, and unfortunately, had to tell them that they did not have the kind of trust that protected anything. They had a revocable living trust that would avoid probate and the court system when one of them became incapacitated or died, but they did not have any kind of asset protection from the costs of nursing home care. Needless to say, this sweet couple was shocked to hear this news, because like many people, they assumed that a trust automatically protected their assets. The truth is that most trusts do not protect any assets at all. They now faced losing a significant amount of their assets that could have been protected with proper advice and planning.

My rule of thumb is that if you can control the assets in a trust, so can your creditors. In other words, if you can take money or real estate out of the trust, your creditors can probably force you to pay them out of those assets as well. If you receive the income from a trust, your creditors can receive that income as well.

If you create the kind of trust that protects your assets, you have to give up some control to get that protection. I have many clients who will create two trusts: one revocable trust to hold things that they want to control for the rest of their lives and a second, irrevocable trust to hold other assets that they want to protect and over which they do not mind giving up control. Sometimes, I have clients who are so concerned about the costs of long-term care that they will give up control over their own home to protect it in an irrevocable trust.

Giving up control, by putting someone else in charge of your home or other assets, can be a hard thing to do. However, if you gain protection from the costs of long-term care, and do not have to worry about the government forcing you to spend most of your estate, or coming after your estate to collect reimbursement for what the government paid for your care after you die, letting a trusted child or other person be the "manager" of those assets can be a small thing to give up in comparison to the great amount of protection you gain from creating an irrevocable trust.

An irrevocable trust can be the best option for people who want to protect themselves and their loved ones from creditors and predators. A creditor may be the state government or nursing home. A predator may be the gold-digger who moves in with your spouse after you have passed away.

Your attorney can draft an irrevocable trust that will protect your assets if you or your spouse require a nursing home. Your attorney can also draft one or more irrevocable trusts to protect assets for your spouse or children when you die. In later chapters, we will explore each of these options in more detail. But first, we will take a look at what long-term care includes and the common options for paying for the costs of long-term care.

# 7
# WHAT IS LONG-TERM CARE?

Long-term care includes a variety of medical and non-medical services for people with chronic illness, disability, or advanced age who cannot care for themselves. Long-term care can be assistance with normal daily tasks like dressing, bathing, meal preparation and using the bathroom, or medical care that requires the expertise of skilled practitioners to address the often multiple chronic conditions associated with older populations. Long-term care can be provided at home, in assisted living, or in nursing homes. People of any age may need long-term care, although it is a common need for senior citizens. By 2020, an estimated 12 million older Americans will need long-term care.

The high cost of long-term care has made planning a critically important issue for most middle class seniors and their families.  In fact, most seniors will likely require some form of long-term care.  Consider these statistics: 70% of Americans who live to age 65 will need long-term care at some time in their lives, and 50% of all couples and 70% of single persons become impoverished within 1 year after entering a nursing home.

Sadly, too many people are unprepared for the significant financial burdens nursing home care places on their family's savings.  Financial devastation looms for a family facing ongoing care at a rate of $10,000 or more per month.

While some seniors are able to afford private pay care, the cost of long-term care will wipe out savings of all but the wealthiest families in a matter of years.  Many people either cannot afford the high cost of long-term care insurance or are not allowed to purchase it at all because of age or medical condition.  If you do have long-term care insurance, you should be aware of what your policy covers.  Many policies have high deductibles or provide for only a short period of care in a facility.  In fact, many people who have long-term care insurance still have to resort to Medicaid to pay for their care. With advanced planning, almost all assets except the family home must be spent before an applicant will qualify for Medicaid assistance.

If the risk of being in a nursing home is that the expense of being there will exhaust all family resources, is there something that can be done ahead of time, before the expense is incurred, to avoid draining the family bank? To understand what can be done ahead of time, you need to have a basic understanding of Medicaid, the program administered by individual state governments and funded by the federal government. Medicaid will pay for nursing home expenses, but only after family resources are exhausted or nearly exhausted.

Medicaid provides medical assistance to low-income individuals, including those who are 65 or older, disabled or blind. Medicaid is the single largest payer of nursing home bills in America and serves as the option of last resort for people who have no other way to finance their long-term care. It is no longer as easy as reviewing one's bank statements to qualify for Medicaid coverage. There are a myriad of regulations involving look-back periods, income caps, transfer penalties and waiting periods to plan around, which we will explore in more detail in later chapters.

The law requires you be impoverished before qualifying for Medicaid assistance, and the quality of care is not what most people would want for themselves or their family member. The fact is, when you go in a nursing home on Medicaid, you will not have the luxury of a personal caregiver to get you to the bathroom. Instead, diapers are the cost-effective, government paid for option. If you want more for yourself or your loved one, you need to plan ahead to cover the costs.

If you do not think you would be able to afford long-term care if you (or your spouse) need assistance in the future, you need to keep in mind that there is some planning you can do to make sure that you are not completely impoverished. The kind of planning that is usually done to prepare for possible Medicaid assistance must be done five or more years before you need long-term care, because advanced planning for Medicaid typically involves a special type of asset protection trust that also protects against probate. We discuss these trusts in detail in a later chapter.

# 8

# LONG-TERM CARE INSURANCE

If you are lucky enough to have long-term care insurance, you have planned for some financial assistance during a period when you would otherwise need to pay heavily for help with your daily living. Failure to purchase long-term care insurance while you are young and healthy can mean that the cost of purchasing it later on will be prohibitive.

Even if you have a long-term care insurance policy, it is best that you take a copy of your policy to an elder law attorney for review, so you understand what it will and will not cover. Most policies only cover certain types of care after a certain period of time has passed and then only up to a certain dollar amount or for a maximum period of time. Making sure you understand the limitations of your insurance will help you understand when it may be time to seek further assistance, such as Medicaid or VA benefits.

Long term care insurance can be an important part of any asset protection plan. The following are some important considerations about these policies.

**Insurance Company Ratings.** You want to purchase a long term care insurance policy from a company that is likely to be around when the long term care services will be needed. While there can be no guarantee that any one of the companies that provide quotes will be there if and when services are required, one factor to consider is the rating assigned to a particular company by various insurance company rating services. In that regard, A.M. Best, Weiss Rating Service, and Standard & Poor's all provide ratings of long term care insurance policies.

**Elimination Period.** The elimination period is a period of time when you may need long-term care, but the insurance will not cover the costs. Elimination periods of 90 days are common. During this time period, even if you need long-term care, you must pay for that care out-of-pocket or from another source. The shorter the elimination period, the higher the premium will be. Conversely, the longer the elimination period, the lower the premium will be. For example, it would be possible to lower the premium on a policy by increasing the elimination period.

**Daily Benefit Amount.** The amount of coverage that a long term care insurance policy provides on a daily basis is called the daily benefit amount. It is usually helpful to look at this amount in the context of a nursing home admission since nursing home costs tend to be the highest of all levels of care (home, assisted living, and nursing home). A typical nursing home can run anywhere from $5,000.00 to $15,000.00 per month, depending on where you live. Therefore, you would need to purchase a daily benefit amount to cover the monthly nursing home costs in your area. While the amount of long-term care insurance alone may be insufficient to cover fully the cost of some nursing homes, when combined with monthly income, there can be sufficient coverage using this daily benefit amount.

**Premium.** The premium can be the single most important factor for an individual who is purchasing long term care insurance. This is a highly personal decision that must take into account the size of the estate as well as the amount of monthly income. Your financial planner and elder law attorney should both assist you in analyzing premium quotes and determining the appropriate level of premiums, given the size of your estate and level of income.

**Level of Care.** There are three levels of care that you will want to be sure are covered under any long term care insurance policy: home and community-based care, assisted living level of care, and skilled nursing facility care. Failure to purchase coverage for all three levels of care could leave the estate exposed in the event that the level of care not covered under the policy is needed.

**Inflation Rider.** It is essential for most people to have some form of inflation protection built into a long term care insurance policy. There are two types of inflation protection that are typically offered: simple (less expensive) and compound (more expensive). Most individuals would benefit from compound inflation protection, unless the person is of sufficiently advanced age so as to warrant simple inflation protection.

# 9
# MEDICAID MYTHS

If you are not one of the few Americans with long-term care insurance, and you do not have sufficient assets to pay the exorbitant costs of caregivers, assisted living, or a nursing home if any of these are needed in your (or a loved one's) future, then, as mentioned above, you may be faced with applying for Medicaid.

Medicaid is the government's plan for paying for health care, including nursing home costs, for people who do not otherwise have a plan to pay for these costs. Unlike Medicare, Medicaid is not based upon a person's age, but rather, on a person's financial need. In other words, the person who would like the Medicaid program to pay for their care will need to be extremely poor.

To be eligible for Medicaid, there are strict requirements for medical need, income levels, and available assets.  Each state has a different, but similar, set of rules to qualify.

Most estate planning attorneys stay away from Medicaid issues. Even judges have a hard time understanding all the legal mumbo-jumbo in the Medicaid rules and regulations. The United States Supreme Court referred to the Medicaid laws as "an aggravated assault on the English language, resistant to attempts to understand it." Another United States appellate court referred to the Medicaid Act as "dense reading of the most tortuous kind."

Needless to say, planning to rely upon Medicaid to pay for long-term care is an area of the law where many seniors need strong, educated guidance to help them figure out the best way to preserve their resources.

One of the most common misconceptions about Medicaid is that a family can just give their assets away before applying for Medicaid.  Giving your property away is a good strategy; the critical issue, however, is the timing of the gifts. The Medicaid administrators will always look at what has been given away over the five years prior to the Medicaid application. Any gift made during that time will result in a penalty period. If you have given away all your assets, and if you cannot qualify for Medicaid because you are in the penalty period, how will you pay the nursing home? There may be some ways to plan around this issue, but the best strategy is to make the gift at least five years before you apply. We will take a look at the best ways to accomplish this, but first, let us dispel some of the Medicaid planning myths you may have "heard" or read about.

The following are some common myths, which are all FALSE:

- Joint accounts will protect assets;
- Putting a child's name on a home will protect the home;
- Giving away all of your assets will protect them;
- Someone in a nursing home must spend down all of his or her assets on nursing home care before qualifying for Medicaid (hint – there are ways to transform and preserve these assets instead);
- It is illegal to transfer assets in the 5 years prior to needing long-term care;
- Once someone is in a nursing home, it is too late to protect assets;
- Medicare will pay for long-term care in a nursing home;
- All powers of attorney are the same;
- A revocable trust will protect assets from Medicaid;
- An irrevocable trust can never be changed or revoked.

We will take a look at some better options to prepare for the possibility that you or a loved one will need long-term care and possibly, the assistance of Medicaid to pay for that care in the next few chapters.

# 10
# QUALIFYING FOR MEDICAID

Currently, in order to qualify for Medicaid, an applicant can have no more than $2,000.00 worth of countable assets. For married applicants, the spouse who is not applying for Medicaid (known as the community spouse) can have up to an additional $123,600.00 of countable assets (subject to potential annual increases), unless increased by a judge's order. This is called the Community Spouse Resource Allowance (CSRA). Available assets are counted toward these limits, and excluded (or exempt) assets are not, as discussed below.

How do you know which assets will be considered available (counted) for Medicaid qualification?

The following assets are available for Medicaid qualification purposes and counted in the asset limit. Please note that for married applicants, Medicaid counts the separate property of both spouses, as well as community property, other joint property, and revocable trust property when evaluating eligibility.

Most assets acquired during the marriage are community property, regardless of whether one or both spouses' names appear on the title. Exceptions to community property include (i) property owned prior to marriage; (ii) inherited property that was not commingled with community property; and (iii) property subject to a transmutation agreement turning the property into the separate property of one of the spouses. But, as stated above, note that the separate property of both spouses is still countable and available for Medicaid qualification purposes.

- Checking accounts;
- Savings accounts;
- Brokerage accounts;
- Certificates of deposit;
- Stocks and bonds;
- U.S. savings bonds;
- Primary residence if applicant does NOT intend to return home;
- Real property, other than primary residence (with certain exceptions);
- Limited partnerships;
- Cash value of life insurance if the total face value of all such policies is greater than $1,500.00;
- Vehicles other than the one excluded vehicle;
- Boats, unless it is your primary residence;

- Recreational vehicles, unless it is your primary residence or your only vehicle;
- Loans payable to the applicant;
- Deferred annuities and some immediate annuities, depending on how they are structured and the date purchased; and
- Retirement funds, generally, but again, there are exceptions and there is always a questions of whether a retirement fund will be considered an available asset or an income stream.

Some assets are specifically excluded (not counted) for determining whether a person is qualified to receive Medicaid benefits. The following assets are excluded for Medicaid qualification purposes and not counted in the asset limit:

- Primary residence if equity is less than or equal to your state's designated allowable equity and the Medicaid applicant intends to return home;
- Primary residence, regardless of equity, if spouse, child under age 21, or a blind or disabled child of any age lives there;
- One vehicle;
- Life insurance with no cash value;
- Life insurance with cash value if the total face value of all such policies is less than or equal to $1,500.00;
- Irrevocable burial contracts;
- $1,500.00 designated for burial expenses (revocable burial contracts, burial savings accounts, or life insurance policies); and
- One burial plot per family member.

A main concern for most families is protecting the family home, especially while one spouse may still be alive and healthy or if a disabled child lives with the person needing Medicaid. As noted above, most state Medicaid rules exclude the Medicaid applicant's primary residence if the applicant is living in the home or intends to return home, and the equity in the home is less than or equal to a certain dollar figure or if a spouse, child under age 21, or a blind or disabled child of any age lives there.

Home equity is calculated by subtracting any debt, such as a mortgage, from the current market value, which is the reasonably expected sales price of the home on the open real estate market. Applicants with an equity interest greater than the state dollar limit are not eligible for long-term care Medicaid (this is known as the home equity cap). The home equity cap may be waived when denial of benefits would result in demonstrated hardship to the applicant.

In most states, the home equity is usually verified by a statement of fair market value from a knowledgeable source and proof of indebtedness. If the home is sold during the Medicaid recipient's lifetime, the proceeds of the sale become an available asset.

While the home may be protected during the Medicaid applicant's lifetime and the lifetime of the applicant's spouse, after the Medicaid recipient's death, if the home is included in the probate estate, then it will be a probate asset subject to creditor claims, including a claim by the state where the applicant was receiving benefits for reimbursement of Medicaid benefits. The state government has the right to place a lien on the Medicaid recipient's home to recover the value of benefits paid, which will be satisfied if the home is sold, whether during the recipient's lifetime or after death. How aggressive this estate recovery process is varies by state.

Certain planning strategies can be used before applying for Medicaid benefits (and after applying for Medicaid benefits in the case of spouses) in order to avoid Medicaid's claim for recovery against the home after the death of the Medicaid recipient, and to prevent the sale of the home from disqualifying the Medicaid recipient from benefits. For example, the home may be transferred to a child caregiver if certain conditions are met, to a disabled child, to the spouse, or to a protective, irrevocable trust. Your elder law attorney will help you decide which option is best for your situation.

# 11
# CRISIS PLANNING VS. PROACTIVE PLANNING

If you are faced with applying for Medicaid for yourself or a loved one, you should consult with an elder law attorney as soon as possible. Do not simply rely on what the government Medicaid workers tell you.

There is an income and a resource (asset) test for people who wish to apply for Medicaid. Your income and your resources cannot be more than the government's set limits. A Medicaid caseworker will review both. If your income or your resources are more than what the government allows, the Medicaid caseworker will deny your request for financial assistance and tell you what portion of your resources (assets) must be "spent down" in order for you or your spouse to qualify for benefits. You certainly can take their advice and simply go out and spend money, but a good elder law attorney will help you figure out the best ways to spend the money while preserving assets and income that is not "counted." The Medicaid caseworkers will not usually give you this kind of advice.

Elder law attorneys will look at all the resources (assets) and the income, and provide you with strategies that may include reducing assets by converting an asset to an income stream. In other words, asset reduction does not have to mean you just give stuff away. Instead, asset reduction focuses on a best use of funds analysis. For example, it may be better to spend money on an asset considered excluded for Medicaid qualification purposes (such as making improvements to your home)? Or it may be better to convert available assets to an income stream (such as purchasing a Medicaid compliant annuity)?

Even in a crisis situation, an elder law attorney can provide essential advice on preserving as much of the estate as possible for the benefit of a spouse or the Medicaid applicant.

Keep in mind that the sooner you plan, the better. Long-term care planning should not be done when someone is in need of long-term care. It should be done while you and your spouse are both healthy and well. This is because the type of planning that can be done well in advance of a person needing to apply for and receive Medicaid is very different from the kind of planning that an elder law attorney can help you with if you need Medicaid at the time you seek the attorney's advice. When someone consults with me at a time when a parent or spouse needs the nursing home, we engage in what I call crisis planning, because we are in the midst of a long-term care crisis and need to take steps immediately to try to protect a spouse or use the Medicaid applicant's funds in a way that will make the most out of their funds. Crisis planning options are much more limited than the options available to clients who are proactive about their planning, and begin the planning well in advance of needing long-term care.

Some tools your elder law attorney may use during crisis planning include: :

- Creation of an income cap trust;
- Purchase of exempt assets, such as prepaid funeral arrangements or a vehicle;
- Creation of caregiver agreements, whereby a relative gets paid for providing care;
- Conversion of countable assets into exempt assets or an income stream;
- Payment of certain debts at the proper time;
- Payment for home improvements.

If money is spent on an exempt asset, such as putting a new roof on the family home or paying off a mortgage, it does not result in any disqualification from Medicaid. If the money is converted to an income stream, it also is not counted as an available asset, but it is counted as income.

It is important to consider all these options and to make the best use of the dollars.

One common way to achieve a spenddown of the available assets and qualify for Medicaid is to pay-off a home mortgage or to spend some money on the cost of renovating or updating the family home. For example, the applicant could spend a portion of the available assets on the cost of an additional bedroom or bathroom for a caregiver, physical changes needed to make the home more suitable to meet its residents' physical disabilities or functional limitations, or to install a wheelchair ramp or chair lift to make entering and exiting the home easier. Other items, such as updating a kitchen, repairing a leaky roof, or purchasing new furniture may also be acceptable for Medicaid spenddown purposes.

This strategy takes assets that would otherwise count for Medicaid purposes, and uses them on an asset that does not count, the home.

Another common planning tool is a family caregiver agreement. If a relative is providing caregiving services to help a loved one avoid living in a nursing home, a personal care contract (also known as a caregiver agreement) could be appropriate. Creating this kind of caregiver agreement avoids the Medicaid office claiming that the applicant just gave money away to a relative. Compensation of a personal caregiver for time and services is an allowable expense for Medicaid purposes if the contract is prepared for future services and the rate of compensation is for fair market value, depending on the level of expertise.

The following are examples of services provided by a relative that may be justifiably compensated under the contract:

- Periodic health assessments;
- Consulting with healthcare providers;
- Securing health care services;
- Monitoring health care providers;
- Periodic assessments of personal needs, supplies, and equipment;
- Visitations;
- Securing social services;

- Shopping for personal hygiene goods and services, clothing, shoes, hobby, and entertainment items;
- Financial management;
- Dealing with others regarding personal affairs;
- Communications with others;
- Addressing resident rights issues;
- Attending to special requests of individual, like dietary requests, or corresponding with family and friends;
- Attending to mail;
- Depositing monthly income;
- Taking individual on trips;
- Taking or arranging for individual to visit friends or relatives;
- Arranging outings, like dinner out; and to
- Prepare and file income tax returns.

The personal care contract is not available in all planning situations. Factors that must be considered when evaluating whether and to what extent a personal care contract may be used include:

- A child caregiver that is providing care on an intermittent and irregular basis;
- A parent or other loved one is of sufficiently advanced age that the life expectancy tables mandate the use of a very short life expectancy (in the case of a large lump-sum payment);
- Extensive assets that cannot be fully spent on caregiver services will require that other planning strategies be used in conjunction with the personal care contract;

- Out of state children caregivers will be more highly scrutinized by Medicaid; and
- Services provided while an individual is residing in a nursing home will be more carefully scrutinized by Medicaid, and in some instances disallowed completely by the Medicaid agency.

As mentioned in an earlier chapter, some people unfortunately believe that they can simply give their assets away and then qualify for Medicaid benefits to pay for their care. Asset transfers (or gifts) for less than fair market value (uncompensated transfers) result in a disqualification period from Medicaid benefits, otherwise known as a transfer penalty period. Under the law of all states except California, there is a 60 month lookback period during which all transfers are reviewed to determine if the transfer or gift was an uncompensated transfer and, if so, what the penalty period will be. If a gift is subject to a penalty period, then the individual who made the gift is not eligible for Medicaid benefits during the resulting penalty period. This 60-month lookback period applies to transfers made to a person or to an irrevocable trust.

If gifts have been made, and the Medicaid office imposes a penalty period, the applicant will be ineligible for a period rounded down to the nearest day. The penalty period may be prorated in the last month so that the applicant may be eligible for only a portion of that month. Medicaid personnel calculate the penalty period by 1) totaling the amount of the uncompensated transfers; 2) dividing the total uncompensated transfers by the monthly average cost of care (nursing home or otherwise) in your state; and

3) the whole number of the result is the number of whole months in the penalty period.

Sometimes, an elder law attorney will advise you to purposefully cause a penalty period by transferring some of the applicant's assets for less than fair market value. Whether this strategy makes sense depends on the numbers, and in particular, whether the applicant has enough money to pay for his or her care during the penalty period.

# 12
# FAMILY PROTECTION TRUSTS

As mentioned in an earlier chapter, some seniors believe that because they created a trust, their assets are protected. The truth is that most trusts do nothing to protect your assets from the costs of healthcare, nursing homes, or other creditors.

Remember: There are many different kinds of trusts.

One of the most popular estate planning trusts, the revocable living trust, is an important part of your estate plan, but it does not protect your assets. A revocable living trust provides an efficient, private plan if you are incapacitated and when you die. They are valuable planning tools, but have significant limitations.

In a revocable living trust, you, and your spouse if you have one, generally act as the trustees (managers) of the trust. You can take any property out of the trust, or put any property in the trust, at any time. You can change who will be in charge of trust and who will inherit the trust assets when you are gone. However, because you can get to your trust assets, a nursing home, or other creditors, can get to your trust assets as well. Because of this ability to spend the trust assets, the revocable trust only provides a very limited form of asset protection: if you become disabled, your backup trustee may be able to step in for you and transfer some of your assets out of the trust to other family members, allowing you to protect a portion of your assets, but these transfers are extremely limited, as we discussed above.

There is another trust option, and that other option is an irrevocable trust. There are different types of irrevocable trusts, some are for wealthier clients who are engaging in asset protection and charitable planning. For now, we will focus on irrevocable trusts that are designed for the average American family. You do not need to be super-wealthy to need asset protection planning. For average families worried about paying for long-term care, there is a trust that will protect your assets.

If a person transfers some of his or her assets to a properly drafted irrevocable trust (what I call a Family Protection Trust), then the assets in the trust will not be available for Medicaid purposes after the expiration of the 60-month lookback period or after any transfer penalty periods have expired, whichever occurs first. When using a Family Protection Trust, instead of just giving your assets to another person, then the penalty period is normally the time period you must wait before the assets in the trust are no longer available for Medicaid purposes. In other words, if you wait to create this trust until you or your spouse needs help paying for long-term care, then anything you transfer to the trust, such as your home, will be identified by the Medicaid office as a gift and used to calculate a penalty period, where the applicant will not receive Medicaid benefits, as we discussed in the last chapter.

With the Family Protection Trust, you are not limited to protecting only half of the assets if you are married. Whether you are married or single, you can protect as many of your assets as you like by planning ahead with this kind of a trust. The irrevocable trust would hold certain assets (such as a brokerage account), and as a result, those assets would not be countable for Medicaid eligibility. However, the assets in the trust would also not be accessible to you, but would be accessible to people that you choose. Those people are called "lifetime beneficiaries" and are often one or more children or close relatives. Upon your death, the trust assets may be distributed to whomever you specified as the beneficiaries in the trust.

The trustee (usually a child, but the trustee can be any trusted person or a corporate fiduciary) manages the trust assets during your lifetime. The person you name as the trustee is only the manager, not the owner of the trust. The trust is the owner of the assets you put in the trust name. The principal cannot be distributed to you under any circumstances, or the trust assets will be deemed an available asset for

Medicaid purposes. The trust is set up in such a way that trust assets can be distributed to the lifetime beneficiaries. The distributed assets clearly belong to the lifetime beneficiaries, and can be used for any purpose that the beneficiaries choose. However, if you name a trusted child to be the trustee (manager) of the trust assets, and put the family farm in the name of the trust, that does not mean the child can sell the family farm or that the child's creditors or ex-spouse can get it. The child can only do what the trust allows the child to do, which in most cases, is to pay you the income from the asset (in our example, the family farm). Another example would be if you chose to put your home in a Family Protection Trust. Your trustee, which may be one of your children, would ordinarily be required to preserve your home for you to live in during your lifetime.

You can even include provisions in these kinds of trusts that will allow you to change who inherits the assets after your death, even though the trust is "irrevocable." One of my favorite sayings is that a good attorney will always find a loophole. And a well-drafted Family Protection Trust is a great example of how loopholes are used. Your irrevocable trust can be dissolved if necessary, and you can even change who inherits from the trust after you die.

Unlike outright gifting, there are several advantages to creating a Family Protection Trust:

- Although the assets are given away, certain rights and powers can be retained.
- The assets in the trust can be protected from the Lifetime Beneficiaries' life circumstances, including: divorce, lawsuits, debts, current or potential creditors, gambling, substance abuse,

disability, undue influence of the beneficiary's spouse and others, financial mismanagement, spending habits, and distribution to a beneficiary's spouse or others upon the beneficiary's death.

- You could receive income from the trust assets, if the trust is so designed.
- You could reserve the right to change who ultimately receives the trust assets upon your death.
- The beneficiaries could get a stepped-up tax basis at your death, if the trust is so designed.

As an example of stepped-up tax basis, assume you purchased an asset for $100,000 that increased in value to $150,000 at your date of death. If the asset were given away during life, the person who received the asset would take it with your tax basis of $100,000. If the recipient of the asset sells it for $150,000 after your death, a capital gains tax must be paid on the $50,000 difference, causing a tax due of $7,500 (at a 15% tax rate). By instead using the trust strategy described above, you can ensure that your heirs take the asset with a tax basis of $150,000, the value at the time of your death. Then if the asset were sold for $150,000, there would be no capital gains and no tax due, saving $7,500.

Because transferring any assets to a Family Protection Trust will require you to give up all right, title, and interest in the assets used to fund the trust, you need to discuss these issues with a skilled elder law attorney. Your discussion should include your cash flow needs, which requires an analysis of your monthly income and expenses, and your comfort level with giving up control of your assets.

Remember that you can pick and choose which assets go to the protective trust and which assets do not. You might choose to keep your home and a small bank account outside the protective trust, as an example.

Keep in mind that assets in a Family Protection Trust will be protected only after a period of 60 months, called the "lookback period." This is a term used by Medicaid as the period in which the agency has the right to review your financial transactions and for you to disclose any transfers made during that period. If transfers were made during that 60-month period, then a transfer penalty, or period of ineligibility, will be assessed by Medicaid. Once 60 months have passed from the date you transfer assets into this trust, the trust might not need to be disclosed (unless an income right was retained) and Medicaid should not assess a penalty—barring any retroactive changes to the law.

If your health fails before the end of the 60-month lookback period, and skilled nursing care is required, you will need to reevaluate your situation at that time. In general, an elder law attorney will consider either collapsing the trust and starting over, or how to pay for your care until 60 months have passed and you can apply for Medicaid. Your options will depend on the law at the time and what can legally be accomplished, but you will always have options.

# 13

# WHAT IF YOU DIE WHILE YOUR SPOUSE IS ON MEDICAID?

Sometimes, one spouse may need Medicaid benefits and live in a nursing home, while the other spouse is healthy and living at home. What happens if the spouse who is not in the nursing home and not on Medicaid dies first? In this situation, the spouse in the nursing home may have been impoverished to qualify for Medicaid, but the other spouse may have more assets that were preserved or income that accumulated in a bank account.

If the spouse in the nursing home inherits these assets from the spouse who died, the spouse in the nursing home will be disqualified from receiving

Medicaid, and will have to spend the inheritance down (possibly the person's second spend down) before going back on Medicaid. This is not necessarily the desired outcome for some couples. Instead, a couple may desire that in such a situation, the inherited assets would be preserved to assist with the nursing home spouse's quality of life. If this is the case, the couple should have created a plan that would take this possible situation into account, and prepared estate planning documents that include a spousal special needs trust.

There is another issue that comes up that creates a special problem if you want to preserve assets for a surviving spouse. In some states, the surviving spouse has a right to a share (the "elective share") of the deceased spouse's estate, regardless of what the deceased spouse put in his or her Last Will and Testament. This is a right to a certain dollar amount, not a right to any specific property. Some of the assets included in the value of the elective estate are:

- The decedent's probate estate;
- The decedent's ownership interest in accounts or securities registered as payable on death, transfer on death, in trust for, or joint tenants with rights of survivorship;
- The decedent's fractional interest in property other than as described above;
- The decedent's revocable trust(s);
- The decedent's interest in any irrevocable transfers in which the decedent retained the right of possession and use of the property;
- The net cash surrender value on life insurance policies on the decedent's life;

- The value of death benefits received under any public or private pension, retirement or deferred compensation plan, other than from the Railroad Retirement Act or from Social Security;
- The value of all property gifted or transferred within one year of the decedent's death, except for property that was sold for full market value; and
- The value of any property transferred in satisfaction of the elective share.

If the surviving spouse is receiving Medicaid benefits and does not make an election to receive his or her elective share amount, some state government offices may consider that a transfer has been made, even though that spouse never received the property. This will result in the surviving spouse being disqualified from receiving Medicaid benefits for a time period calculated by dividing the value of the unclaimed elective share amount by the state-determined monthly cost of nursing home care.

The flip side to this situation is if the surviving spouse claims the elective share, he or she will be over the Medicaid asset limit and will be disqualified from further Medicaid benefits until the elective share funds have been spent down to under $2,000.00.

You should consult with an elder law attorney both before and upon the death of a spouse so as to ensure that the surviving spouse's Medicaid benefits can be dealt with appropriately, and the maximum amount of assets can be preserved.

Despite whether you live in a state where the elective share amount must be distributed to the surviving spouse, any amount remaining in the decedent's estate after satisfaction of the elective share can still be directed into a supplemental needs trust (more on these later!) for the benefit of the surviving spouse in order to maintain the surviving spouse's Medicaid benefits. The trustee of the supplemental needs trust can use the trust assets to pay for any items or services not covered by Medicaid. Another option is for the remaining assets to go to other non-spouse beneficiaries, such as children, other relatives, or charities.

If you believe that you or your spouse face the possibility that you will be reliant upon Medicaid to cover the costs of your long-term care in the future, it is important to address some steps you can take in your estate planning documents to protect each other as much as possible should one of you die first.

# 14
# SPECIAL BENEFITS FOR VETERANS

Many wartime veterans and their surviving spouses are currently receiving long-term care or will need some type of long-term care in the near future. While these veterans can apply for Medicaid if financial assistance is needed, the Veterans Administration (VA) has funds that are available to help pay for this care, yet many families are not even aware that these benefits exist. The benefits are referred to as pension, aid and attendance, and housebound benefits.

A veteran may be eligible for pension with an additional award for aid and attendance if certain service, income, asset, and medical conditions are met:

- The veteran served at least 90 days of active military service, 1 day of which was during a wartime period; or if the Veteran entered active duty after September 7, 1980, and served at least 24 months or the full period for which called or ordered to active duty (there are exceptions to this rule), 1 day of which was during a wartime period; and
- The veteran was discharged from service under conditions other than dishonorable; and
- The veteran's countable family income is below a yearly limit set by law (the yearly limit on income is set by Congress); and
- The veteran does not have an excessive net worth; and
- The veteran is age 65 or older or permanently and totally disabled, and now requires the assistance of another person as explained more fully below.

A surviving spouse of a wartime veteran may be eligible for a benefit called death pension with an additional award for aid and attendance if the deceased veteran met the wartime, active duty and discharge requirements above, the surviving spouse has limited income and assets, and is over 65 or disabled and requires the assistance of another person as explained more fully below.

As noted above, there are income and asset limits that must be met before a veteran or spouse can receive these benefits. Countable income is income received by the veteran and his or her dependents, if any, from most sources, including earnings, disability and retirement payments, interest and dividends, and net income from farming or a business. For VA pension eligibility purposes, a dependent includes a spouse, so the income of the veteran and spouse are included as countable income.

Net worth means the net value of the assets of the veteran and his or her dependents. It includes assets such as bank accounts, stocks, bonds, mutual funds, and any property other than the veteran's residence and a reasonable lot area. There is no set limit on how much net worth a veteran and his dependents can have, but net worth cannot be excessive. The decision as to whether a claimant's net worth is excessive depends on the facts of each individual case. All net worth must be reported, and the VA will determine if a claimant's assets are sufficiently large that the claimant could live off these assets for a reasonable period of time. The VA's needs-based programs are not intended to protect substantial assets or build up an estate for the benefit of heirs.

It is possible to reduce assets and income to a level that will be acceptable to the VA. For example, excess liquid assets (such as cash or stocks) could be converted to an income stream through the use of an annuity or promissory note. However, because the claimant may need to qualify for Medicaid in the future, it is critical that any restructuring or gifting of assets be done in a way that will not jeopardize or delay Medicaid benefits. Like Medicaid benefits, veterans benefits are also subject to a look-back period and penalty period if gifts are made within three years of applying for benefits. An attorney who has experience with elder law will be able to provide valuable assistance with this.

Once an application is submitted, it often takes the VA more than a year to make a decision. Once approved, benefits are paid retroactively to the month after the application was submitted. Having proper documentation (discharge papers, medical evidence, proof of medical expenses, death certificate, marriage certificate and a properly completed application) when the application is submitted can greatly reduce the processing time.

In order to calculate the pension amount, you will need to total all countable income. Then subtract any out-of-pocket recurring medical expenses. The remaining countable income is deducted from the appropriate annual pension limit, which is determined by the number of dependents, if any, and whether or not the veteran is entitled to housebound or aid and attendance benefits. This amount is then divided by 12 and rounded down to the nearest dollar. This gives you the amount of the monthly payment.

Aid and attendance (A&A) and housebound are benefits paid in addition to monthly pension. These benefits may not be paid without eligibility for pension. Entitlement to A&A benefits exists when the claimant requires the aid of another person in order to perform personal functions required in everyday living, such as bathing, feeding, dressing, attending to the wants of nature, adjusting prosthetic devices, or protecting himself or herself from the hazards of his or her daily living environment. The veteran may receive this benefit when he or she is bedridden, a patient in a nursing home due to mental or physical incapacity, or is blind. Housebound benefits are for veterans who are permanently and substantially confined to their immediate premises due to medical disability. The VA will consider a claim for housebound benefits if a veteran is denied aid and attendance benefits.

The Veterans Administration will provide nursing home care if the veteran meets any of the following criteria:

- The Veteran requires nursing home care for a service-connected condition; or
- The service-connected disability rating is 70 percent or more; or
- The service-connected disability rating is 60 percent or more and the Veteran is not employable.

The VA may provide nursing home care to veterans who do not meet the above criteria if space and resources are available. Veterans who have a service-connected disability are given first priority for nursing home care.

To find information on applying for these benefits, go online to "www.va.gov" and select "Benefits," then "Compensation and Pension." You have the option of filing an application online or printing an application and submitting it yourself. This site will provide you with the appropriate forms and explanation for filing a claim. You may also call the Veterans Administration toll-free number (800-827-1000). And, finally, an attorney accredited by the VA can assist you.

# 15

# SELECTING TRUSTEES: DON'T TRUST YOUR CHILDREN JUST BECAUSE THEY'RE YOUR CHILDREN

Whether you create a will, power of attorney, or a trust, trusting the wrong people is a common estate planning mistake.  Many people believe that it is the "right thing to do" to name a family member to manage their affairs if they are no longer able to do so.  Not only do people tend to name family members, but they will name children to manage their estate in an order based upon age. These decisions are not always made because they are well-reasoned, sound decisions. Instead, they are made because "that's how it's always been done." The decision to name a family member is often an emotional, rather than a logical, decision.

In a similar way, children will try to fulfill their designated role because they feel obligated to do so. The truth is, most children are too busy and lack the skills to make financial and health care decisions for aging parents or to administer an estate or trust when a parent dies. Our world is a very fast-paced, busy place, where kids have plenty to do on a daily basis trying to keep their own lives on track. The designation as a trustee, personal representative (executor), or agent under a power of attorney or health care power of attorney can be too much to handle for some children or other family relatives.

Naming a child or other relative simply because they are related to you or because you believe they should take care of you as you age can be fraught with more severe problems. In an extreme circumstance, I became involved in a case where an elderly man lived in a nursing home, had a $2,000,000.00 estate at the time he moved into the nursing home, and had "planned" his affairs by naming his only son on his power of attorney. Why would the DA be getting a call about this elderly man? Because senior services became involved when the man was given notice that he was about to be evicted from the nursing home for failure to pay his nursing home bill. Apparently, the only son had liquidated his father's property and spent it . . . on himself. This son left his father penniless and a victim of the court system, as he needed to have a professional guardian and conservator appointed to make decisions for him for the rest of his life, given the failure of his only child to properly care for him. This man, who had the financial means if it had been properly managed to pay for his nursing home from his own funds for the rest of his life, wound up on Medicaid and moved to a different home where Medicaid patients were accepted, instead of the private pay, more luxurious home in which he had been living.

In another case, my client's son filed a petition with the local court to be appointed my 90 year old client's (his mom's) guardian and conservator – in other words, he was attempting to prove that his mom could no longer make her own decisions due to her age, that he should be allowed to move her into a rest home, and move himself and his new girlfriend into his mom's beautiful, lake-view house. It turned out that this mom was smarter than her son, and she proved to the court that she was perfectly capable of making her own decisions – including the one to disinherit her son. These cases show that despite our desires to the contrary, kids can have their own, rather than their parents', best interests in mind and behave in very selfish ways.

Children are not the only ones who can be poor choices to control you and your assets if you are incapacitated or to manage your estate when you die. Trusting the government can be worse than trusting your children. One senior who came across my criminal case load was a victim because he had no planning, friends, or family and was relying on the state office for seniors to send a caretaker to assist him. It was discovered that this man had "gifted" his government-supplied caretaker over $16,000.00. She was, of course, prosecuted and convicted of felony theft.

My point with these true stories is that if you are going to create an estate plan, choosing who your decision-makers will be is often the most important decision you will make during the estate planning process. It is not uncommon for this decision to also be the hardest one to make.

Here are a few things to consider along the path of reaching your decision:

- Do you have any children who are 100% trustworthy to carry our your wishes in your best interest?
- Do those trusted children have the time and ability to manage your finances and your healthcare as well as their own?
- If you do not wish to name children or do not wish to name children, would any other relatives be desirable and capable?
- If you have a blended family, do you and your spouse agree on a single child, or do you wish to name a child or another person from each of your "sides" of the family to act jointly?
- If you do not like the idea of any of your kids, relatives, or friends managing your affairs, have you considered a corporate fiduciary, such as a bank or other professional?

I have taught workshops where we discuss the pros and cons of naming different types of trustees in estate planning documents. A clear winner is often a professional, such as a bank, accountant, or other professional fiduciary to manage a client's finances.

While you may not like the idea of not having a family member whom you personally know and love carry out your wishes when the time comes, professional trustees are often the best choice because they eliminate the emotion, they know how to administer a trust or estate, and are for that reason, extremely cost-effective and efficient. They also more easily stand-up to any family members who might otherwise push around the child or relative you leave in charge. This last point can be a particularly important consideration in blended families, or in a situation where you are leaving assets to a troubled child.

# 16
# DON'T MAKE YOUR HUSBAND'S NEW WIFE (AND HER KIDS) RICH!

The next story is about an estate planning case I became involved in that turned murder-mystery: A man remarried in his 80s to a woman 30 years his junior. The man wanted to include his wife in his estate plan, and specifically left her the house they were living in and all its contents, plus some cash accounts. Although his estate plan left everything in the home to his wife, he trusted her to distribute sentimental items to his children without specifically writing this intent in his trust. He left other property and investment accounts to his surviving children. When this man died (less than one year after marrying his young bride), his wife had a storage unit ready. She moved everything out of the house they had been living in, including the family photographs of his children and other sentimental heirlooms. The kids did not receive any of these items. This woman threw property in a dumpster she had parked in front of the house rather than give it to the children who would have cherished the items. After a bit of investigation, we learned that this same woman had been married eight times previously, and had done a similar dance upon each husband's death.

In other cases, I have seen estate planning documents that simply leave everything to the surviving spouse. While this may be your wish, what if your spouse outlives you, remarries, and then leaves the entire estate to the new partner? This happens quite frequently, leaving kids with no ability to request anything (such as photographs) from a parent's belongings. If you leave everything to your spouse without any kind of restrictions, your spouse owns those items upon your death. Your spouse can then remarry and create a new will or trust that leaves everything to the new person. Think about that new partner then leaving everything you left to your spouse to his or her own kids, and your own, biological children wind up with nothing. Some simple restrictions and agreements between you and your spouse while planning your estate can prevent this from happening.

The blended family situation is a modern estate planning concern. One of the most common lawsuits after someone dies is between the person's biological children and the new spouse. If you are in a blended family, and do not leave a very clear and up-to-date plan in place, you can be certain that your loved ones will have disagreements. These disagreements may be resolved between them through compromise or fought out in the court system.

With some couples, the marriage may begin with a valid prenuptial agreement, which the couple follows for the first few years of their marriage, keeping assets titled in "his" and "her" names. When these marriages last, and a spouse does not die until years down the road, children and the surviving spouse may realize that the dead spouse's intentions were not left entirely clear. Prenuptial agreements are frequently ignored after a number of years of marriage. For example, the couple may agree to leave retirement plans to each other, but not use the required language in their prenuptial agreement when they name each other as pay-on-death beneficiaries on these accounts. This leaves the door wide open to children fighting with the new spouse about enforcing the prenuptial agreement and disregarding the pay-on-death beneficiary designations.

I have personally seen this happen, and have seen the intended spouse lose in court because the prenuptial agreement was never formally dissolved, and the court will choose to enforce it. When a spouse dies, the court does not care what a husband told his wife before he died or vice versa. The court cares about what the couple agreed to in writing, and can choose to protect the biological children instead of the surviving spouse.

While you may need to make sure you do not unintentionally disinherit your biological children by leaving everything to your spouse, who then remarries and leaves everything to the new partner, you similarly need to make sure you do not unintentionally fail to plan for your surviving spouse, if it is your desire to do so. Both sides of the blended family situation should be thoroughly discussed, and your intentions made clear in a well thought-out estate plan.

# 17
# DON'T MAKE YOUR EX SON-IN-LAW RICH!

I internally cringe when someone wants to include an "in-law" as a successor trustee, personal representative (executor), agent, or beneficiary in their estate planning documents. Do not get me wrong. I find it refreshing when families get along, and especially when the love extends beyond the biological members. The problem with giving in-laws any power in your plan is that statistically, they too often become out-laws. When they leave the family, they are still named in your plan unless you can, and do, remove them. Of course, by now you know I have a story to tell. On this topic, I have plenty of stories. But there is one that stands out.

After a man's father died, the man realized a crucial mistake in his father's estate plan. His dad was a widower and had prepared a living trust with a lawyer's assistance. The dad did not want to overburden his busy son and knew that his daughter-in-law frequently took care of the personal, family business, such as paying the bills. The dad was under the impression that his son and daughter-in-law had a loving relationship. The trust named the daughter-in-law as the trustee (manager) of the estate after the dad died, and if he became incapacitated. The trust also left half of the estate to the daughter-in-law. When the dad became incapacitated, the daughter-in-law agreed to step in as his successor trustee, as the trust requested, to manage the dad's affairs. From that point forward, this daughter-in-law controlled the dad's bank accounts and all of his property. Unknown to the son and his father, she was also having an affair and began stealing from her father-in-law's trust accounts. In fact, she stole over $100,000.00 from his trust bank account by the time the son found out. The dad died shortly after all of this came to light. The son reported the crime to the police, but the case was not filed in court, because the dad (the victim of the crime) had died and, of course, could not testify, so law enforcement felt the case was too weak.

So, the son was left in a difficult position, because he knew what his now ex-wife had done, but there was no criminal conviction for the elder abuse and theft. He was left with the option of going to the probate judge to request that his ex-wife be removed, even though law enforcement had not filed criminal charges against her. Here's the point: if you are incapacitated or die, it becomes difficult or even impossible to change your plan to match the change in your in-laws.

My recommendation is not to name in-laws in your estate planning documents. If you do, make sure your attorney includes a statement that if the in-law is soon to be an out-law because one spouse has filed for divorce or separation, or the couple is no longer living together as a husband and wife, that the gift or appointment as a trustee, agent, or personal representative is null and void. The man in the above example failed to include this very important provision, which could have avoided the awful situation he left for his son.

# 18

# PROTECTING YOUR KIDS FROM PREDATORS, THEMSELVES, & THEIR SPOUSES

Your planning focus will likely differ depending on whether you have young children or adult children. Protecting adult children who are spendthrifts, in and out of prison, in precarious marriages, or who simply have different philosophical belief-systems than you can be an important part of your plan. Most parents, once they realize they can leave an inheritance in a protective trust for their adult children, are excited to do so. Even if your adult children are wonderful, responsible people, leaving their inheritance in a protective trust that the child can manage will at least gives them a choice about whether to leave the funds in their protected trust or spend the money.

For adult children, much can also be written in a trust to restrict how the children can spend the funds. For example, you could create a trust for a child that would give your trustee the ability to tell a drug-addicted child "no," or that the child may only receive trust money if the child completes a substance abuse treatment or rehabilitation program, or to hold funds if a child is in prison. You can even put restrictions on how the money is spent, such as not allowing the child to donate any portion of his or her inheritance to charities whose philosophical beliefs are different from your own.

For example, consider a Catholic couple who love their only son very much, but the son is married to a man and heavily supports the charities that contradict his parents' beliefs, such as "Planned Parenthood." While the parents may still desire to leave this son a substantial portion of their estate, they may prefer to leave it in a way that he would have a large retirement income, but would not be allowed to simply donate the funds to his charitable causes.

In contrast, when kids are younger, parents will often choose to "motivate" them to attend college, or start a business, or otherwise accomplish some life goals before the child receives any substantial money from a trust. This planning can be necessary to avoid the "trust-baby" syndrome that can strike wealthier kids who receive a large inheritance. Trust distributions can be broken up or limited to an annual amount, to ensure that the child does not just blow through the funds. A sum of money can be given upon completing college, or at an older age if college is not completed, to motivate a child to get a college education and realize a monetary reward.

Decades ago, attorneys would frequently draft these "educational trusts" in a way that required the trustee to cover the costs of the education and also to give the child a certain percentage or fraction of the trust at certain ages. For example, the trust might say that upon reaching age 25 or upon completing a college education, the trustee would give the child 1/3 of the trust funds, and then another 1/3 upon reaching age 30, and the remaining balance at age 35.

Modern estate planning attorneys tend to steer away from such forced distributions, because the money that is required to be distributed is available to creditors the child may have at the time. A good estate planning attorney will take this possibility into consideration, and suggest to you that a better way to draft a trust for a minor child may be to allow the child to step in as the trustee or a co-trustee and manage the trust funds at a certain age. This way, the trust funds can remain in a protected trust, and the child can spend the money however you allow them to in the trust, but creditors cannot force the child to give them the money.

Planning for minor children involves more than simply planning for money management, because you must also address who will raise your children. Naming a guardian for minor children has nothing to do with setting up a manager for any assets you may leave behind. It is easy for parents to put off estate planning, because they do not think they have substantial assets to protect. This outlook is common among young adults, who think they have plenty of time to accumulate wealth and plan for it at a later date. However, in failing to create a proper estate plan, many parents do not adequately protect their children. All parents, with or without a great deal of assets, should have an estate plan in place to set forth their wishes for their children and the nomination of a guardian in the event that they have an untimely passing while the child is still a minor.

Even parents who make some effort to plan by naming their choice for a guardian often fail to leave any specific guidance for their children and the guardian. This specific guidance should be left in a written document that spells out the parents' life philosophies, hopes for their children, and their wishes for the children's schooling and religious upbringing.

If there is no plan in place, the court will appoint a guardian to raise your children based on what the court deems to be in the best interest of your children. Unfortunately, the court-appointed guardian may not be your first choice, and in some cases, he or she may actually be your last choice. From just a few brief hearings, it is often impossible for the court to determine who is best-suited to care for your children in your absence. In some cases, where no clear-cut guardian is named, children may be sent to child protective services to remain with a foster family until the court decides on a suitable guardian to take on the responsibility. For many parents, this scenario is reason enough to create an estate plan to protect their children.

Nominating a guardian can be a very difficult decision. The individual selected should provide stability for your children in the difficult transition and ultimately continue care in a fashion with which you are comfortable.

You should consider the following traits and circumstances when determining who is best suited to raise your children:

- Age: You will want to make sure the guardian is old enough to provide proper care (at least 18 years of age in most states) but young enough to remain in good health until your children reach adulthood.
- Commitment: Ensure that the guardian does in fact want to take on this responsibility.
- Temperaments: Carefully consider what kind of person will mesh well with your children. If you have young or energetic children, you may want to make sure the guardian exhibits patience.
- Religious and moral beliefs: Do they share the same values as you and your spouse? Would they instill these in your children?
- Nature of existing relationship with children: You will want to make sure that this person has a good bond with your children and that there is a mutual comfort level.
- Location: If you prefer that your children not move out of their current home or school district, you will want to make sure that the appointed guardian resides close to you and

intends to stay there until your child reaches the age of majority.

- Does the proposed guardian have other children? If so, does the guardian have enough time and resources to devote to their own children in addition to yours?
- Finances: Can the candidate financially provide for your child if there are not enough funds available from your estate?

In the event that the guardian you have selected in your estate plan is unable to raise your children upon your passing, you should have at least one alternate who also meets your criteria. This will ensure that your children are left in the hands of trusted relatives or friends and not in the court system. If you have children and would like to appoint different guardians to raise them separately, you may also outline more than one guardian appointment in your estate plan, but this situation is generally not regarded as ideal for close siblings. All appointed guardians must ultimately be approved by the court at the time of the parents' passing.

Another modern problem is our society's divorce rate, and the existence of biological parents who are estranged from their children. If a biological parent is still living, they will usually be named the guardian of the children unless evidence is presented that this individual is unfit to provide care to the children in question.

All parents of minor children should create a trust that is designed to safeguard the inheritance for their children. Such a trust gives you the ability to outline how much money your children will receive, the age at which they will receive the inheritance and to an extent, how they are to spend this money. This allows you to designate funds for their college educations and give them their inheritance at a certain age, ensuring that they don't waste their inheritance on fancy cars as soon as they turn eighteen years old. As mentioned above, the trust can also protect against potential creditors or even divorce. Trust funds can also be used to provide support to your children until they reach the age at which they may receive their inheritance.

In your estate plan, you must also name a trustee who can ensure this money is handled properly. The trustee may be different from the guardian selected in your estate plan. A different person or entity who will serve as the trustee is a good idea if the guardian is good with children but not with money. Having a trustee who is not also serving as the guardian provides a "check and balance" system, which can help ensure that a guardian does not spend the money selfishly (such as for an unnecessary, new house or new furniture) rather than preserving the funds for your children.

Trusts also allow you to protect both your spouse and your children by dividing your assets between them, so if your spouse is not wise with money or remarries, your children will still be protected. A trust allows you to outline how the trustee is to budget funds for each child. If you have one child who has a special need or requires additional training to develop a talent, your trust may outline these appropriations. This is particularly important if you have a child with physical or mental disabilities who may require significant care throughout his or her entire life.

Children are often the greatest assets that parents have and an integral part of the estate planning process. Your children's well-being is only ensured with proper planning and, while most parents hate to think about leaving their children before they are adults, it is essential that this possibility be considered and an effective plan formulated.

# 19

# PROTECTING A DISABLED LOVED ONE WITH A SPECIAL NEEDS TRUST

If you have a family member with special needs, you face some unique challenges and issues of concern.

For example, how can you leave an inheritance to a loved one without jeopardizing the special needs person's eligibility for the means-tested government benefits available?

How can you design a plan that supplements the government benefits and enhances the life quality of the special needs person?

How do you equitably treat other children in the family when doing this planning?

How do you provide proper supervision for any funds you leave for the care of the disabled loved one?

If you have a child or another loved one who is physically, mentally, or developmentally disabled, he or she may be entitled to government benefits such as SSI or Medicaid. Most benefits are available only to those with limited financial assets and income. As a result, leaving an inheritance to a disabled loved one may cause the loved one to no longer qualify for government benefits. I have been involved in cases where an inheritance was left to a disabled person who tried to refuse the inheritance, because the disabled person would lose needed government benefits by receiving extra funds. The problem that comes up in these scenarios is that even when the disabled person refuses the inheritance, the government still counts it received, even though the disabled person never actually received a dime. The act of refusing money the disabled person could have received is enough to cause the government to deny benefits.

Is there a way to allow such a family member to receive an inheritance and also continue to receive government benefits? The answer is, "yes."

A special kind of trust called a "Special Needs Trust" (also called a Supplemental Needs Trust) can be drafted to supplement government benefits by providing only benefits or luxuries above and beyond the benefits the disabled person receives from any local, state, federal, or private agency. A special needs trust designates a trustee, who will have complete control over the distribution of assets and income to the beneficiary. The beneficiary of a special needs trust cannot have the right to demand any principal or interest from the trust.

The special needs trust is designed to supplement (which is why these trusts are also called supplemental needs trusts), rather than replace, government assistance. Assets placed in a properly designed special needs trust do not belong to the beneficiary, so they will not disqualify him or her from Medicaid or SSI benefits. You can fund the trust during life or at death using a variety of assets, including cash, stock, real estate or life insurance proceeds.

To preserve eligibility for government benefits, trust funds must not be used for the disabled person's support. In other words, they should not be used for medical care, food, clothing, or shelter covered by Medicaid or SSI. But they can be used for just about anything the government does not pay for, including rehabilitation and medical care not covered by public benefits, education and training, transportation, insurance, wheelchair-accessible vans, and modifications to the disabled person's home. A special needs trust also can be used to pay for quality-of-life expenses, such as travel, recreation, hobbies, entertainment, and stereo and television equipment.

Each state has different rules regarding a person's ability to qualify for government benefits. Therefore, it is imperative that you consult with an estate planning attorney who is well versed in drafting special needs trusts in the state where your beneficiary is receiving government benefits. Special needs trusts are a powerful estate planning tactic which allow you to make sure that your loved one is well cared for after you are gone. You will have peace of mind knowing that your child or other beneficiary will not only be able to continue to receive benefits, but can also enjoy an inheritance that provides them the lifestyle you would choose for them if you were still living.

In my office, we include an optional special needs trust in every estate planning trust we prepare. This optional special needs trust can be used for any beneficiary named in the trust. That person may not be disabled at the time the trust was created, but may be later on. The optional special needs trust ensures that everyone included in the estate plan is protected, no matter what life may bring in the future.

# 20
# DON'T LET "FLUFFY" BE EUTHANIZED

One of the main goals of estate planning is to provide for your loved ones, and for many of us, "loved ones" includes at least one pet animal. While you can always ask a friend or relative to look out for your pet, they are not legally obligated to do so unless you set up an estate plan for your pet. If you do not have a plan that quickly and easily provides for your pet's food, shelter, and care, you should consider creating one.

The way the law views animals makes it critical to choose the right planning method. Even though you consider your pet as a companion and devoted friend, legally, your pet is considered "personal property" and is not given the status of a person. The specific estate planning method you use will depend on your state's laws, your pet's needs, your goals, and your financial resources. Working together, you and your attorney can plan for the best method to ensure that your pet will continue to have a quality life.

You could provide for your pet in your last will and testament or by creating a trust.

Even though it may seem "easy" to include a bequest for your pet within your will, it may not be the best approach, for the same reason we discussed avoiding will-based planning in earlier chapters. Your will must go through probate before it takes effect. This can be time consuming and uncertain, and your pet will need immediate attention. Your pet is not like your spouse, adult children, or your siblings – they can take care of themselves until the probate process is complete.

But since your pet needs food, water, shelter, and love every day, this may not be the best way to provide for your pet. During probate, your pet's care, or even ownership, can be in jeopardy. So, while you may want to include provisions in your will for your pet, first consider other methods. Many people are now using a "pet trust" to provide funds and direction for the care of their pet.

Unlike a will that is subject to the probate process, a trust becomes effective immediately upon the terms outlined in your trust – usually death or disability. Your trust specifies the details concerning the care and control of your pet, as well as making funds available. Your trust can also give specific directions about the daily care, medical attention, physical control, and even burial of your pet.

Like other trusts, a pet trust is a legal entity set up to accomplish a particular purpose. You and your attorney will outline the specifics that detail when and under what circumstances the trust will take effect. This includes how the trust will be funded, who will be the trustee, successor trustee, beneficiary, and caretaker, and how the trustee or caretaker will manage your pet and the funds for your pet. You want your pet to be fed, cared for, and to receive medical attention. You may also want to designate funds for pet insurance, or even to enforce the trust. In your trust, you can also leave real property for housing your animals.

A "pet trust" is a generic term and is applied to any trust that provides for your pet. A pet cannot be a beneficiary of a traditional legal trust, because one of the legal requirements for a trust is that there must be a beneficiary, and that beneficiary must be able to enforce the terms of the trust. Obviously, a pet cannot enforce a trust. So, the choice and structure of a trust must take this into account and be properly worded to accomplish your goals.

Some states have passed laws that allow for enforceable pet trusts. These laws allow the trust creator to designate a third party who will have the power to enforce the terms of the trust – to force the caretaker or trustee to use the trust funds for your pet.

An "honorary trust" is a type of trust set up for a specific purpose (such as to provide for a pet) but without a definite beneficiary. The problem with an honorary trust is that without a state law specifically authorizing it as a pet trust, it is essentially unenforceable.

One of the best methods to ensure the care of your animals is to set up a traditional legal trust. Your attorney can carefully add language to avoid problems. One method used is to place the pet and sufficient funds into the trust. The pet and the funds are the body of the trust. Your attorney then names the caretaker of your pet as the "beneficiary" of the trust. You name a trustee – the party responsible for managing the funds and the caretaker. Having a trustee who is different from the caretaker will create a "check and balance" system to ensure the caretaker does not withdraw all the funds from the trust for themselves, rather than spending the money on your pet.

How much money you leave in the trust depends upon your finances, your pet, and the amount of care that will likely be involved for the pet's anticipated life span. Obviously, providing for the care of some pets will be more expensive than for others. If your pet is an elderly dog, you will not need to designate as much money as you would for a young horse.

# 21
# THE FAMILY FARM: PASSING & PROTECTING YOUR LEGACY

Estate planning for farmers and ranchers poses unique challenges. The family farm is a personal legacy, which has often been in the family for generations. Emotional attachments to the farm can be strong. According to the USDA, approximately 97% of the two million American farms are family owned. Family farms account for the largest percentage of the value of all farm production, having a critical impact on the rural economy. The average

age of a farm operator is 57, and the fastest growing operator segment is over age 65.

Despite the aging farm owner population, most farmers have not planned to pass the family farm and do not have a succession or estate plan in place. The conversation can be hard to have with family members, because farm owners often foresee problems with a future transition, both financial and emotional. However, once the family farm owner's concerns are known, a creative estate lawyer will be able to provide viable solutions.

A frequent problem with family farm planning is that some children are involved, or wish to be involved, in the farming operation and some children do not. Parents often do not want one child to receive a greater gift than the other children. The family lawyer must craft a transition that considers the non-farming children. Fair does not necessarily mean equal, and dividing ownership of the farm equally between all children is usually a recipe for disaster. Sometimes, the farm owner can simply gift to non-farming children from another area of the family's wealth; for example, life insurance. If other assets are not available, a farm operations limited liability company, which allows farm-involved children to have managerial duties and a salary, as well as a distribution from profits, and uninvolved children to receive a smaller distribution as their share of the inheritance, can be a good option. These creative solutions will prevent a forced sale of the land, which may be required to pay taxes and distribute the property to the children in accordance with state law if no planning is accomplished.

To begin the farm planning process, I meet with my clients to construct the family history and to understand the family hierarchy and the relationships between siblings, parents and children. I learn of each family member's strengths, weaknesses, state of marriages, and ability to handle finances. The role played by each person, their educational background, sacrifices made, including the long, hard hours worked, are all taken into consideration. I also obtain a detailed description and analysis of the current farming operation, including a sketch of the acreage, how each parcel relates to the other, identifying roadways and various houses on the farm. It is not unusual for more than one family member to live on the farmland or for the farm to be the family's most sentimental family legacy.

Taking the situation and goals into consideration, I, along with other team members, usually a certified public accountant, a financial advisor, an insurance professional, and a banker, develop a strategy that coincides with the farm owner's objectives.

Failure to plan can cause financial problems for both the farm owner and the potential successor, be a source of family conflict, and result in the forced sale of land to pay taxes or other obligations. Proper planning, will instead allow the farm to endure, while caring for the needs of both generations.

# 22
# DON'T MAKE YOUR FAMILY INTO FELONS WITH YOUR FIREARMS

Many issues can arise when a gun owner dies, leaving firearms behind. I have witnessed family members commit felonies because of the way they have collected, transferred, and possessed these left-behind family heirlooms. While you may see a firearm as your grandad's favorite pistol, the law sees it as a deadly weapon that is regulated to the point of defying common sense. There are so many rules and restrictions pertaining to who can possess firearms, how you can lawfully transfer them, and how you can carry or transport them (especially when moving them across state lines), that most people, even people who own many guns, do not understand these laws. If you wish to learn more about these many gun-control laws, please read my book, *Infringed*, which spells out, in plain English, the many rules and regulations that control how you can possess, transport, transfer, and use firearms. Violation of any of the gun-related laws is a criminal offense, meaning that the people who break these laws can face jail time, probation, and loss of their gun rights.

Firearms in estates or trusts must be analyzed by addressing all applicable state and federal laws.

When a gun owner dies, the first question should always be whether the firearms are secure. If the owner has died, did that person leave a firearm (possibly loaded) where others (possibly inexperienced people who do not know anything about guns) have access to it? The firearms should be stored in a way where only the person who will administer the estate or trust (assuming that person is not prohibited from possessing firearms under any laws) will have possession of them, and also a place that will make theft unlikely.

If a person in charge of an estate or trust does not secure the firearms, that person can be sued for negligent entrustment or even charged with a crime if the wrong person gets possession of the firearm.

Once the firearms are secured, the second inquiry must be who can be in lawful possession of the firearms. When a person dies, the court usually appoints a personal representative (also called an executor or executrix) to take control of all the estate assets. The personal representative can legally transfer the firearms to other people or sell them. If a gun owner dies after transferring all of his or her firearms to a gun trust (more on these later), the gun trust should designate a successor trustee, and that successor trustee can lawfully possess the firearms without any action by a court. If the personal representative or the successor trustee is a prohibited person (cannot legally possess firearms), then another person must be designated to possess and transfer the firearms to the intended recipients.

The next inquiry is to determine what types of firearms the person owned, and whether any of them were illegally owned. Some firearms require registration in a national registry (required by a law known as the National Firearms Act or "NFA") regardless of your state of residency. These firearms are referred to as "NFA Firearms." If the owner of one of these firearms dies, it is unlawful for anyone to possess them unless the owner previously made arrangements through a trust or named someone in a will as the personal representative for the estate (for a "reasonable time") until the court has issued an order giving a specific person legal authority to possess them. Violating these rules is a federal felony that carries a potential ten-year prison sentence.

In addition, many states now have regulations that require the registration of additional firearms, or that ban many types of firearms that may have been legal where the gun owner lived and died. These state laws prohibit these illegal firearms from crossing state lines into the state that bans them, even if they were legal for the dead gun owner to have in his or her state.

If you are in charge of an estate as a personal representative or a trustee for the person who died, you must determine whether the estate includes any

NFA firearms and if so, to whom they are registered. If you are unable to locate any paperwork showing the registered owner, then the personal representative of an estate can request this information from the federal Bureau of Alcohol, Tobacco, Firearms and Explosives (the "ATF") in writing. When you make this written request to the ATF, you will have to disclose your identity and the identity of the firearm in question. If the estate owns unregistered NFA firearms, the unregistered NFA firearms cannot be possessed or transferred. The personal representative for the estate should immediately contact the ATF and arrange for disposal of any unregistered NFA firearms, as it is not legal for the personal representative to remain in possession of them. If the firearm was illegal for the original owner to possess, then it is illegal for anyone else to possess. The person delivering contraband to the ATF is shielded from prosecution. If you have additional questions, it would be a good idea to contact a firearms attorney.

If the NFA firearms are properly registered, there is still paperwork to be completed and approved prior to transferring the firearms. It is not uncommon for an unsuspecting spouse to possess NFA firearms unknowingly. You should also make sure that any transfers will comply with the laws of any of the states in which the firearms will wind up.

If the estate assets include firearms that are not NFA firearms, then all of the laws and rules about possession and transfer must be addressed. There are too many such laws to address them all in this context. The person in charge of the estate or trust must determine whether any heirs are prohibited from possessing firearms. If so, then such a prohibited person cannot receive their inheritance. Before transferring any firearms in an estate, you must check ages and the laws of the states where the heirs live. Different states have different age requirements for firearms, and those age requirements sometimes depend on the type of firearm. Some firearms are prohibited in certain states, and obviously, you cannot transfer firearms to a state where they are not allowed.

The best practice, before transferring firearms in an estate, would be to use the services of a federal firearms licensee (FFL) or at least require a copy of the heir's concealed carry permit. Remember that some states require that an FFL be used to conduct a background check before any transfer can take place, and some states require registration of certain firearms.

I help many gun owners create a "gun trust" to ensure that their loved ones are aware of the firearms and how to manage them when the gun owner becomes incapacitated or dies. A gun trust is a special type of trust that is designed to hold all of your firearms and firearms-related accessories. A well-drafted gun trust will prevent many of the problems that family members run into when they inherit firearms, or when the gun owner simply becomes incapacitated.

When properly written, gun trusts are powerful asset protection and estate planning tools. A well-drafted gun trust will achieve the following for the gun owner who creates the trust:

- Ensure that friends and family can lawfully possess and transfer trust-owned firearms during the gun owner's lifetime;

- Create a private plan that completely avoids the court system for all firearms if the gun owner becomes incapacitated or dies;
- Helps the successors and heirs to understand the gun owner's desires related to all the trust-owned firearms;
- Helps the ones you care about to comply with firearms laws when they possess or transfer the firearms;
- Assists the gun owner to own firearms in more than one state; and
- Ensures that neither the gun owner nor any loved ones commit an accidental felony.

The following stories illustrate how things can go wrong when firearms are not properly addressed in an estate plan.

A widowed father created a generic last will and testament online. He wrote in the form that he wished to leave his entire firearms collection to his beloved son. Unfortunately, by the time the father passed away, the son had been convicted of a domestic violence offense. The father never updated his last will and testament, and he did not know enough to leave an alternate plan for the firearms in the online form, or even to simply state that if for some reason one of his heirs could not receive a specific gift outlined in the will, the heir would receive something else in place of the specific gift (such as stating that if his son could not receive the firearms or the firearms no longer existed at the time of his death, that the son would receive cash or some other property of similar value in place of the firearms).

The father also wrote in the form that he wished

for his other child, his responsible, hard-working daughter, to act as his personal representative.

Like many children, the daughter and her brother met at their dad's home after his death to divide his personal belongings. During that process, the daughter gave all of the guns to her brother, and he drove them back to his home in California.

The daughter and her prior lawyers did not have a clue that she and her brother broke the law. Gun laws do not always require that the violator have knowledge of the criminal law violation for charges to be filed. The poorly drafted will in this situation left no alternative gift to the son, did not name an alternate beneficiary to receive the guns, and did not in any way address the laws pertaining to the possession or transfer of the firearms.

This scenario is a classic example of an "accidental felony." The daughter knew her brother was convicted of a domestic violence offense, but did not understand the laws enough to refrain from giving him guns. Her behavior is typical of many children inheriting firearms from their parents—they do not know enough to stop and think about all the rules they must obey when transferring the guns to the intended recipients.

In another case, an aging wife was concerned about her husband's declining mental capacity due to Alzheimer's. She was worried about being able to manage their affairs on her own, because his retirement plan administrator denied her access to information on her husband's separate retirement account when she called to ask a few questions. The couple never completed any estate planning documents—no will, no trust, no power of attorney, no health care directive. This woman's husband had a gun collection that included NFA firearms. She was never interested in firearms, had no idea of their value, and would have preferred to have nothing to do with any guns (except to sell them so she could have more money to care for her husband). She took a couple of the full-autos (machine guns) to a gun shop for an appraisal, but was asked to leave, because she did not know anything about the paperwork they were requesting to see. By the mere act of taking these machine guns to a store, the wife committed an "accidental felony" by unlawfully possessing and attempting to transfer the machine guns.

The husband, in this example, was the only person who could be in lawful possession of the machine guns. For the wife to have lawful possession, she needed to proceed to court and ask the judge to appoint her as her husband's legal conservator in order to avoid committing a crime by simply holding the firearms. If the wife made this request to the court, and the judge appointed her or another person as her husband's conservator, the husband will be "adjudicated a mental defective" and will not be able to legally possess any firearms anywhere in the United States. The wife will either need to transfer all of the firearms out of the home or, at a minimum, lock them in a safe and not tell her husband the safe combination.

Let us take a look at how a properly drafted gun trust would address the above situations.

When someone has a well-written gun trust, the people named in the trust to manage property if the creator of the trust dies or becomes incapacitated, will have a wealth of information available to them in the trust document itself. My gun trusts read like books, and my clients often comment on how much they have learned about gun laws simply by reading their trusts. Because all this information is in the trust itself, the successor trustee will be alerted to many issues that can create potential civil and criminal liability. We will assume for the remainder of our discussion that the gun trust that could have been created for the people in my examples was well written and that it included all the things a competent firearms attorney would include in the trust.

If the father in my example above had created a gun trust instead of a last will and testament, these accidental felonies would have likely been avoided. The trust would have, in black and white, prohibited the transfer to the son and alerted any attorney and the personal representative to his status as a "prohibited person" because of the domestic violence conviction. The trust would have clearly outlined who "prohibited persons" are under both state and federal law. There would have been no question that the son could not have legally received the firearms. In other words, the criminal behavior would have been completely avoided.

The trust also would have made it clear that the son was not entitled to any substitute assets in lieu of the firearms, to eliminate any fighting amongst the remaining heirs. The trust would have directed that the guns go to the father's alternate beneficiary (the daughter) to sell or keep, depending on her wishes. The firearms would also not be listed in any public court proceeding, because firearms owned by a gun trust do not need to be "probated" when the creator of the trust dies. Whoever received the firearms would have been able to receive them quickly, efficiently, and without court paperwork or a public record.

A gun trust would also have saved the wife in my second example from needing to go to court to be able to legally sell her husband's guns. When a spouse becomes incapacitated, the other spouse's primary concern is usually to care for the incapacitated spouse. The typical secondary concern is how to come up with the financial means to do so. The last thing a person in this situation wants to do is pay an attorney to assist with a court process, have his or her spouse ruled by the court to be mentally incompetent, and invest the time, energy, money, and stress involved in all aspects of filing a court proceeding. A well-planned gun trust could prevent this situation from occurring simply by making the wife a trustee or beneficiary of the trust.

With a gun trust, the need for a guardian or conservator with respect to the firearms would have been completely eliminated, and there would be no fear of violating any laws if the wife decided to take some time to keep the firearms in the home, sell them one by one to achieve top dollar, or transfer them to other people. The gun trust would have given her complete legal authority to do whatever she needed to do (or what the gun trust dictated she should do), such as give the guns to children, grandchildren, friends, or any other named beneficiaries in the trust. Again, the court system, the delays, and the fear of violating the laws, would have all been eliminated with a properly prepared gun trust.

As you can see, gun trusts have invaluable benefits over no plan or even a will-based plan. Trust planning in general provides a more seamless plan for incapacity and death, and in the realm of firearms, it is by far superior, because a gun trust specifically addresses the firearms laws.

When clients create a will-based plan, they often also sign a "Durable Power of Attorney," where they name someone to act on their behalf if they are incapacitated. Any firearms law-related provisions are almost always entirely missing from these documents. A gun trust will cure issues related to named agents' or trustees' lack of knowledge about your guns and gun laws and will prevent them from committing an accidental felony. Like other trusts, gun trusts are also usually private, and they avoid guardianships, conservatorships, and after-death probate.

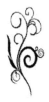

# 23
# THE DANGERS OF REDNECK ESTATE PLANNING

When one of my clients was diagnosed with cancer, his doctor advised him that his odds of survival were not good. In a quick effort to make sure his sons did not have to go through probate, he went to the county courthouse to sign a deed so his two sons would inherit his home. Or so he thought.

The county clerk assisted him by telling him that if he added his sons to his deed "with right of survivorship," his sons would inherit his house when he died, and a probate proceeding would not be necessary.

One year later, this man was still alive, had a new girlfriend, and wanted to refinance his home with the Veterans Administration. When the bank told him that the other owners (his sons) would have to sign the mortgage paperwork, he was shocked. He was even more surprised when he asked his sons to sign off on the title to his home, and they refused.

My firm wound up filing a lawsuit to remove the sons from the deed to this man's house. We had to prove to the court that this client had no intention of giving his sons any ownership interest in his home when he signed that deed. While the clerk at the courthouse was correct that the boys may have become the sole owners of the property when this client died without having to go through a probate, she failed to advise the man that this type of "planning" is fraught with problems. A major problem with adding other people to the deed to your home or as a joint owner on a bank account is that if you put a child's name on a deed, or a bank account, or on the title to any other assets, that child now has an ownership interest in that property . . . and so may the child's creditors, including a divorcing spouse.

Which brings me to my next story. Another client of mine put her daughter's name as joint owner with right of survivorship on her checking and savings accounts. This was, according to my client, intended to serve two purposes: 1) the daughter could manage the money if she became ill or otherwise incapacitated; and 2) the daughter would simply inherit what was left in the account when she died, without having to endure a probate proceeding. Unfortunately, the daughter found herself involved in a heated divorce, and the soon to be ex-husband was so malicious that he claimed part-ownership in ALL accounts that had his wife's name on them – including her mom's joint account. At the end of the day, we won the case for my client, but she had to endure the stress of this unnecessary and completely avoidable hassle.

It is easy to think that you can avoid attorneys, expensive fees, and probate simply by placing a child's name on the title to an asset. However, there are severe problems that arise when conducting this kind of "estate planning." I refer to this kind of planning as "redneck estate planning," because of people's effort to make such vital decisions without professional advice in an effort to avoid the perceived expense of hiring a professional.

The situations I described above are just a couple that can arise with redneck estate planning. This type of planning often does not even accomplish the intended goal, to avoid probate, because if any children or other natural heirs are excluded, they often claim that the parent or other person who added a child's name to an account did not intend to gift an interest in the account, but merely put a child on the asset as a convenience so the child could help out the parent or other person.

For example, if an aging widow in her 90s, who has three children, but puts only two of these three children on a bank account, the third, left-out child will likely argue to a court that the widow put the two children on the account so they could help her pay her bills. In other words, the mom merely put the children's names on the accounts to help her out in her old age rather than intending to give the money to those children to take out for themselves while she was still alive. In many courts, all the left-out child needs to prove is that the original account-holder (in my example, the mom), did not intend to allow the added children to take the money to spend on themselves while she was alive, but only after her death. These lawsuits are often an emotional and financial drain for the family members who have to endure them.

Some people may not name a child as a joint owner on an account, but may instead use "pay-on-death" beneficiary designations to name the children or other people who should inherit assets when they die. Some significant assets, including life insurance policies, retirement plans, and even bank accounts, allow a beneficiary to be named in this manner. Naming pay-on-death beneficiaries is free, easy, and, when the owner of these accounts dies, these assets are designed to be paid directly to the person named as beneficiary, outside of probate.

Unfortunately, there can still be significant issues with this type of planning. For example, if the person you name to inherit is under 18 or incapacitated (disabled) when you die, the court will most likely take control of the funds. This is because most life insurance companies and other financial institutions will not knowingly issue payment to a minor or an incompetent person, nor will they pay to another person for the child, not even to a parent. They do not want the potential liability and will usually require proof of a court-supervised guardianship or conservatorship. They will insist on this court supervision. I have been involved in cases where the financial institution demanded a court-appointed conservator for a minor, even when the minor's parents are still married and living together and raising the child. The financial institution does not want to get sued later by the child, when the parents have spent the money for themselves, instead of preserving it for the child when he or she turns 18.

If you name "my estate" as your beneficiary on these assets, you are requiring a probate. This is because the financial institution will now require a personal representative appointed by the probate court to receive the funds on behalf of the estate and be responsible for getting the funds to your heirs or the people you named in your will. In other words, the funds will have to go through probate, so they can be distributed along with your other assets.

If your beneficiary dies before you (or you both die at the same time) and you have not named an alternate beneficiary, the proceeds will have to go through probate so they can be distributed with the rest of your assets to your surviving, lawful heirs.

Even in cases where the funds are paid to the named beneficiary, things may not work out as you intended. For example, some people cannot manage large sums of money. They may spend money irresponsibly, be influenced by a spouse or friend, make bad investment choices, or lose the money to an ex-spouse or creditor. If the beneficiary receives a tax-deferred account, he or she may decide to "cash out" and negate your careful planning for continued long-term tax-deferred growth.

If you name someone as a beneficiary with the "understanding" that the funds will be used to care for another or will be "held" until a later time, you have no guarantee that will happen. This trusted person may become incapacitated or die, leaving your intended funds to their own family and heirs.

If the person you name as beneficiary is receiving government benefits (for example, a child or parent who requires special care), you could be jeopardizing their ability to continue to receive these benefits.

If your estate is on the larger side, your choice of beneficiary could limit your tax planning options, causing serious tax consequences for your family.

My point is that beneficiary designations can be quite useful, but they need to be considered as part of an overall estate plan rather than the sole means of avoiding probate. Naming a trust as beneficiary will generally prevent the problems described above, and by bringing all of your assets together under one plan, you can be sure that each beneficiary will receive the amount you wish for them to receive—something that can be difficult to accomplish with multiple pay-on-death beneficiary designations.

As you can see, what many people think will be a simple solution to their estate planning problems is often the cause of lawsuits and fighting amongst family members in court.

# 24
# PREVENTING ELDER ABUSE

Elder abuse can be mental, emotional, or physical. A client once told me that she lived in a senior mobile home park, and she sometimes received telephone calls from people who asked if she signed her own checks as soon as she answered the phone. These callers were clearly thieves, targeting seniors, and looking for easy money. These thieves can escape prosecution for a long time, as they fabricate stories about why a senior wrote them a check, such as to repay them for work they did around their home, or to buy groceries. These wretched criminals sometimes make a good living preying on their vulnerable victims.

Elder abuse can also be much more technologically sophisticated, such as "pop-up" questions on a computer. The unsuspecting seniors answer questions that pop up on the internet about their bank accounts, only to find out they have given someone money or access to their account.

One way to stop financial elder abuse is to make sure you do not give out your financial information to anyone. Seniors, or their concerned family members, can also set limits on daily spending on credit and debit cards and receive a text or email notification every time money is debited from an account. Another option is to lock credit, so that no one can apply for credit or open a financial account in the senior's name.

Credit protection companies, such as LifeLock, are well worth the monthly fee, because they will alert you if anyone applies for credit in your name.

If someone tells you that you owe them money, do not be afraid to ask for a receipt. Also ask for identification from people who knock on your door. Better yet, do not answer your door to strangers, do not answer questions strangers may ask you, and do not answer your telephone if you do not recognize the caller.

Every state has a government office that focuses on the elderly and can investigate allegations of abuse. If you or someone you know is being abused, you should check if your state laws provide for a special restraining order for seniors.

If your state has an elder abuse restraining order, the information is often on-line or even available in paper form at the local courthouse. The packet will describe your state's requirements for obtaining a restraining order. Make sure you qualify for a restraining order by reading the eligibility requirements. The packet also includes the forms you must complete to request a hearing. If you do not have an attorney to help you complete the packet, you may be able to obtain help by contacting your District Attorney Victim Assistance Office.

If you are completing the forms on your own, be sure to read the instructions carefully, and complete the forms as instructed. If you make a mistake, you may not be able to obtain the restraining order. Once you have reviewed and completed the forms, you must file them with the court clerk. There is usually no fee to request a restraining order. The clerk will then set a hearing date for you to appear before the judge.

The court may be required to set a hearing on your request for a restraining order very quickly, usually by the next business day. If the judge decides that you are eligible for a restraining order, the court will issue the order. The order must be served on the person who abused you. Service is usually accomplished by the court clerk delivering a copy of the restraining order to the Sheriff and requesting that the order be personally served on the person abusing you. Check with the court clerk if you are unsure of the procedure in your area. The order will be in effect for one year.

After the abuser has been served with a copy of the restraining order, he or she may request a hearing. The abuser may present evidence at the hearing, and may even hire a lawyer to present his or her side of the story. You should strongly consider hiring an elder law attorney at this stage if you have not done so already. Not all abusers request a hearing; however, if such a hearing is requested in your case, you must appear and present your case as well, or the judge may change or cancel the restraining order based on the evidence presented at this second hearing.

If the abuser violates any provision of the restraining order, you should contact law enforcement immediately and report the behavior. Violation of a restraining order can result in the abuser being arrested, charged with contempt of court, and punished by jail time and a fine.

The best option to avoid elder abuse is to plan ahead by having your trusted people in place to protect you if you become victimized. If you do not have a plan and are victimized, then a restraining order can be a great solution if available in your state. If your state does not have a restraining order, then you may still be able to file a court case, either based on an elder abuse law in your state or through the criminal court system, by making a complaint to law enforcement.

An experienced elder law attorney can help you determine if you may be eligible for a restraining order, complete the required application for a restraining order, report the abuse to law enforcement, and make sure that your rights are protected. An elder law attorney can also assist you by filing a complaint for elder abuse to recover property taken from you or to request damages related to the abuse. If your request for a restraining order is contested (meaning the abuser asks for a hearing), an elder law attorney will present your case to the judge by questioning witnesses, presenting other evidence such as photographs or documents, and making legal arguments on your behalf.

Regardless of your financial worth, the potential for fraud and abuse exists. This is why a well-drafted, comprehensive estate plan will include a plan for your incapacity that leaves your trusted people in control of your health care and finances. A properly drafted incapacity plan prevents elder abuse because it directs certain people to manage your finances in a specific manner, and because it does not allow others to benefit from your money.

Although planning for incapacity is an essential part of creating an estate plan, I often find it is the most neglected aspect of a client's plan. For example, living trusts often do not even define the word "incapacity," leaving those who must decipher the document with an avenue for argument.

Many seniors do not have a trust, and are instead relying on an outdated, incomplete, or worse, an overly-comprehensive power of attorney. Some clients only have a will, often drafted using a software program instead of competent legal advice, which cannot under any circumstances address a client's care during their incapacity. The prevention of elder abuse starts with a good estate plan that fully addresses who will step in, and when, if the creator of the plan is ever incapacitated.

# 25
# TWO DOCUMENTS THAT CAN REDUCE YOUR RISK OF ELDER ABUSE

Estate planning can involve a few, or many, different documents. Depending on your personal situation, a knowledgeable estate planning attorney will create a custom plan tailored to you, by using trusts (revocable or irrevocable), wills, personal property memorandums, powers of attorney, advance health care directives, HIPPA release documents, and business succession planning documents such as buy-sell agreements. More complex estate plans may include entities such as limited liability companies or corporations, family foundations, and charitable gifting through special, charitable trusts.

These documents may address incapacity, death, or both, but if you ask a friend or family member what the phrase "estate planning" means, they usually will not even mention any planning for incapacity, but will most often tell you it means a plan to pass their belongings after they die. As we saw in the last chapter, instead of creating a will or a trust, many people try to get around the probate or trust system by naming beneficiaries on accounts, or worse, adding their kids as joint owners on the title to their assets.

As we also saw in the prior chapters, if you add another person to the title of your assets, you have given up control. The newly added owner, and their creditors, now have rights. Bankruptcy, divorce, the unforeseen judgment creditor, can now claim and sometimes take what was once yours. If unrestricted in these designations, children can also use your money to take care of themselves, instead of you. After all, when you put them on your accounts, did you intend to give them the money? If you cannot speak for yourself, what would the child who took the money say?

There are better ways to make sure that someone you trust can help you if you need their assistance. Preparing a couple of inexpensive documents while you are able to plan ahead can help you avoid falling prey to abuse without giving up control as described in the above situations.

There are two documents that everyone should create, regardless of the size of the estate: a health care directive and a financial power of attorney. These documents become your voice when the crisis happens, and can help you avoid a guardian or conservator being appointed on your behalf. Because your named, trusted agents can take control upon your incapacity, preparing these documents can help you avoid being a victim.

**Health Care Power of Attorney & Living Will or Advance Directive**. Depending on where you live, these documents may be called a living will and powers of attorney for health care, a living will, or an advance directive. Whether you are rich or poor, it is imperative that you name your trusted medical decision-maker. The person you name to make medical decisions for you is called your health care "agent."

The health care durable power of attorney allows you to name a person to make medical decisions for you if you become incapacitated. When your healthcare agent is called upon, he or she is entitled to consult with health care providers for informed consent, to have access to appropriate clinical records, and to apply for benefits such as Medicare and Medicaid.

It is important to discuss your wishes about future medical decisions, life support systems, and artificial nutrition and hydration with your healthcare agent. You need to inform them of the location of the original copy of your health care durable power of attorney. You should also speak with your doctor and other health care providers about your wishes. Upon entering the hospital or other health care facility, you or your healthcare agent will need to provide copies of your health care durable power of attorney to the admissions staff.

The living will specifically limits the scope of treatment, including the withholding of tubes for food and water, if such treatment is futile and against your wishes. It limits the scope of medical treatment if you become comatose, suffer from a chronic terminal illness, or are in a persistent vegetative state. It is very important for you to speak with your doctor concerning your wishes regarding life-prolonging procedures.

If you are living in an assisted living facility or nursing home, you need to ask them about their policy in regard to living wills and do not resuscitate orders (DNRs) and plan accordingly.

If you have any reservations about family members (children, siblings, parents) fulfilling this role, you should act immediately. If you do not have close family members to fulfill this role, you should still designate your preferred person (neighbor, friend), rather than allowing the court to appoint a "professional" guardian.

Health care powers of attorney and living wills can be customized to include:

- Your religious beliefs (Jehovah Witness, LDS, Jewish, Catholic, etc.)
- Special provisions if you experience dementia
- How to address your agent if he or she objects to your direction to remove life support or tube feeding
- To supply human contact if you are dying
- Maximizing pain and anxiety relief
- Expressing your wishes regarding autopsy
- Compensating your health care agent

- Your desire for home care over an assisted living facility
- Naming an agent for your children
- Addressing your desire to receive alternative treatments such as acupuncture, chiropractic care, and massage
- Address whether life support or tube feeding provisions apply if you are pregnant
- These provisions are usually not included in standard advance directive forms, but if they are important to you, you should express your wishes in the written document and bind your trusted agent to carry out your wishes.

**Durable Power of Attorney.** A durable power of attorney gives the person you choose (your Agent) the legal authority to handle all of your financial matters. This authority may be limited in any way you wish. The durable power of attorney is effective once signed and remains in effect until you die or choose to revoke it. If you become ill, your Agent will be able to manage your financial affairs. There should be no need for a court to declare you incompetent or to appoint someone to manage your financial affairs. If you are declared incompetent by a court, then the court's authority could override that of the durable power of attorney. Too often, powers of attorney documents are inadequate for one of two reasons: 1) they are too broad, granting an agent too much power; or 2) they are too limited, in that the document fails to grant a power that is needed. A power of attorney can fail, because it may contain standard, "form" language, that allows your only child to spend your money for his or her own benefit. If questioned, the child might claim that you intended for him or her to do so to avoid estate taxes. A power of attorney can also fail, requiring a court to appoint a conservator, when it does not specifically give your named person the power to complete a specific task, such as filing for Medicaid or preparing a trust for your benefit, or to transfer your property to a trust that you already created. The people involved in the transaction that your named agent is trying to accomplish for you (such as the Medicaid office or a title company) may refuse to accept the power of attorney, and insist on a court order.

There is a 65% chance that each of us will experience some period of incapacity during our lifetime and a 10% chance of suffering a period of incapacity lasting longer than one year. Planning with a durable power of attorney and your state's health care documents is vital to avoiding a conservatorship or guardianship proceeding, and can save your loved ones thousands of dollars in attorney fees and court costs.

# 26
# WHAT ABOUT ESTATE TAXES?

Unless your state imposes an inheritance or estate (death) tax, most people do not have an estate that is taxable after Congress passed President Trump's tax reform in 2017. An individual in 2019 can pass an estate worth $11.4 million dollars without worrying about any federal estate tax. Beware, though, that some states collect a tax upon a person's death on estates worth as little as one million dollars, so you need to consult with an estate planning attorney in the state where you live or where you have property to fully understand if your estate requires tax planning.

If you have accumulated substantial wealth during your lifetime, and, as a result, face estate tax issues, you should consider special planning to preserve your estate for your heirs to the greatest possible extent. A well-advised client will utilize special tools, such as tax planning in their living trusts, family asset protection trusts, family limited liability companies, dynasty trusts, life insurance trusts, and charitable trusts, to ensure that their wealth is passed to their intended beneficiaries in a manner that decreases taxes and protects assets from creditors and predators.

If your estate is taxable, federal tax law allows an unlimited transfer of property to a surviving spouse without imposing any estate tax. This is a result of what is called the "unlimited marital deduction." In addition to the unlimited marital deduction, federal tax law allows every individual to transfer a specific amount tax-free during his or her lifetime, or at death, to a beneficiary or beneficiaries other than a spouse. This amount is called the "exclusion amount." Some states simply follow the federal law; others impose a tax on an amount less than the federal exclusion amount, which, again, is why it is imperative that you consult with an estate planning attorney in your state.

If you are married and leave everything to your spouse without proper tax planning, then upon your death, your estate will not have to pay any federal estate taxes due to the effect of the unlimited marital deduction. But when your spouse dies, all amounts in excess of the exclusion amount will be subject to both federal and state tax rates.

For example, let us assume you and your spouse have a combined taxable estate of $30,000,000 (note that your taxable estate usually includes everything you own or have control over – including life insurance proceeds – at the time of your death). If you were to die in the year 2019 leaving everything to your spouse, no federal estate taxes would be due at that time. If your spouse then were to die in the year 2020, the first $11,400,000 (which will be updated annually for inflation) would pass free of federal estate tax, but the remaining amount would be taxed, unless your accountant makes a portability election or you have otherwise planned to use both exemptions.

A simple, basic way to avoid or minimize this tax problem for married couples is to establish an estate plan that creates a new trust when the first spouse dies: a "Family Trust" (also called a "Credit Shelter Trust" or "Bypass Trust"). The purpose of the Family Trust is to provide support for the surviving spouse during his or her lifetime, with the remainder of the trust then going to the children upon the death of the surviving spouse.

Using the above example, upon your death, at least half of your estate would be left to a Family Trust instead of directly to your spouse. Your spouse could be the trustee of the trust and would be allowed to receive all the income from the trust every year. Your spouse can even withdraw additional principal from the Family Trust, so long as the money withdrawn is not used by your spouse to exceed the standard of living established while you were alive.

Upon the death of your spouse, the Family Trust will terminate, and whatever is left in the Family Trust will go to your children – completely free of estate tax, even if the amount they receive has grown to be more than the amount that went into the trust at the time of your death.

Because the tax laws now allow what is called a "portability" election, which essentially accomplishes the same tax savings that this type of Family Trust planning accomplishes, it is not always necessary to use this type of trust planning to achieve the tax savings. However, many couples choose to use this type of trust planning simply to protect a portion of the trust assets from the issues that can arise when one spouse dies first, and the surviving spouse remarries, as we saw in prior chapters. This type of trust planning can be used whether or not you have an estate that is over the exclusion amount. Some couples worth much less than the exclusion amount will create this type of trust planning for asset protection instead of tax protection.

# 27
# QUESTIONS TO ASK YOUR ESTATE PLANNING ATTORNEY

Choosing the lawyer who will guide you through the estate planning process is an extremely important decision. You should not choose a lawyer simply because their office is conveniently located, you are friends with or related to the lawyer or the lawyer's family, or, especially, because they are cheap. While these are certainly valid concerns, none of them should be the sole basis for your selection. The number of years someone has been a lawyer may not even be a good indicator of their estate planning expertise. Some lawyers may have been practicing law for 20 years or more, but may have only drafted a few estate plans a year. Other lawyers, who focus on estate planning as a specialty, may have drafted thousands of estate plans.

A good estate planning attorney will easily be able to tell you how many trusts and wills they have drafted. They can also tell you how often they have been involved in probate proceedings and administering trusts after the trust creator has died or become incapacitated. Lawyers who have experience with the family feuds that they are trying to avoid for their clients are better estate planners, because of their experiences. They know where the problems lie, and will work with you to specifically address the problem areas in your family dynamics or in your estate.

Lawyers who specialize in estate planning and elder law are almost always members of national groups where they can attend special educational classes and collaborate with other estate planning and elder law attorneys. Lawyers in these groups share their experiences and help each other with problem cases through their collaboration. A young lawyer with little experience requires mentoring to gain experience. You do not want a new lawyer to gain their experience by making a mistake with your plan.

Do not be afraid to ask your lawyer questions. Do not be afraid to leave and get second or even third opinions before you hire someone.

Your lawyer should also be able to tell you how they justify their fee in the estate planning documents they create for you. If you meet with a lawyer who charges twice as much as another lawyer down the road, ask them what is different or special about their estate planning documents. I can list for my clients what I do in my trust documents that other lawyers frequently leave out. I even provide my prospective clients with a chart that shows the difference between my plans, online forms, and other, common, lawyer-drafted plans.

Ask your prospective lawyer if they have any experience with your particular family issues – young kids, adult problem children, charitable distributions, farms and ranches, special needs trusts, irrevocable trust planning, Medicaid, seniors, or gun owners. If you are a veteran and wish to learn more about veterans' benefits, make sure the lawyer is accredited with the VA, which is required before the lawyer is able to advise you about veterans' benefits. You want to know if the lawyer has the expertise at the time you hire him or her. You probably are not interested in the lawyer who says they have little or no experience with your important issues, but they can "look it up."

Ask the lawyer what they include in the power of attorney and the pour-over will. Will they include provisions to protect your spouse if you die and your spouse is on Medicaid? Will they include protective trusts for your children? Will they include a stand-by special needs trust that can be used if any of your named beneficiaries becomes disabled before you die? In what ways will their documents protect a surviving spouse or biological children in a blended family situation? Will they help you "fund" the trust by titling your assets in the trust name? Does the power of attorney include any special powers related to Medicaid planning and income cap trusts?

The bottom line is that you should not be afraid to ask and make sure the lawyer you are hiring has the credentials, experience, expertise and ethics to help you.

# 28

# THE PITFALLS OF PARALEGALS AND DO-IT-YOURSELF PLANS

With the number of online and do-it-yourself (DIY) legal providers continuing to grow, some readers may be wondering if they could create their estate planning documents themselves. The advertising is seductive: attorneys use similar forms, the cost is significantly less than hiring an attorney, and many of these websites and kits are created by attorneys. In addition, most people think their estates are not complicated, and many think they are just as smart as (or smarter than) professionals.

Creating a legal document without legal advice is risky business. All you need to do is read the disclaimers posted by internet sites or software companies selling innocent people what are supposed to be legal forms – these disclaimers almost always advise you that the company selling the form 1) is not a lawyer; 2) cannot give you legal advice; and 3) that you should have legal advice. These disclaimers usually finish with a statement that the company is not responsible for anything. In other words, the company selling you a cheap form is telling you "don't use our software – go see an attorney." And for good reason – fill-in-the-blank forms cannot replace solid legal advice. If you create your own estate plan incorrectly, there is no malpractice insurance company that will come to your aid. Attorneys are educated, have your best interest in mind, and are insured if they make a mistake. There simply is no substitute for solid, professional advice when creating an estate plan.

During the 20 years I have practiced law, I have yet to review a do-it-yourself form that was filled out properly. After speaking with clients about what they intended to write on the form, they most often did not spell out their intentions correctly. One of the most common mistakes is to fail to plan for contingencies. It is easy to fill out a form and indicate that you wish for your estate to be divided equally amongst your surviving children. Most people, however, list all of their children without specifying what percentage each child should receive. Should each child get an equal share? If you do not specify this in the document, it is left unclear. But what if one of your children dies with or before you? What if one of your children suffers an accident that leaves that child incapacitated? A good estate planning attorney will think in layers, and plan for important contingencies (the "what if" situations).

Most professionals know that DIY estate planning can be very dangerous. While completing the forms may seem easy and straightforward, a single mistake or omission can have far reaching complications that only come to light after the person has died. With that person not here to explain his or her intentions, the heirs could end up disappointed and confused, and could end up paying much more in legal help to try to sort things out after the fact than it would have cost for a lawyer to prepare the plan in the first place. A judge I became acquainted with early in my career (and who became a good friend and mentor), told me that attorneys make money not by planning, but by cleaning up the messes. This judge was right. One will contest will easily net my firm ten times the cost of drafting a trust.

If you are considering drafting your own will or trust, consider the following:

Legal Expertise: Experienced estate planning attorneys have the technical expertise to draft documents correctly. Yes, they may use pre-drafted forms to start from, but they know what to change and how to change it to make your plan work the way you want. They also understand the technical terms and legal requirements in your state. Laws vary greatly from state to state, and a DIY program or kit may not tell you everything you need to know to prevent your plan from being thrown out by the court.

Counseling: Attorneys are called "counselors at law" for a reason. Most estate planning attorneys have counseled many families, and they have seen the results of proper and improper planning. One of the most important things I do for my clients is to provide them with options and opinions. During my initial consultations with clients, they frequently say, "I never thought of that." That is, of course, the point of being in my office. An experienced attorney will bring up all aspects of your plan, and make you think about the things you had not previously considered. The attorney can guide you with delicate decisions, including who should be the guardian of your minor children; how to provide for a child or elderly parent who has special needs without interrupting valuable government benefits; how to provide for your children fairly (which may not be equally); and how to protect an inheritance from creditors and irresponsible spending.

Explanation of Intentions: If there is any confusion as to what your intentions were after you are gone, the attorney who counseled you will be able to explain them. This unbiased interpretation from someone who does not stand to benefit from your plan can help to avoid costly litigation by your beneficiaries and even maintain the validity of your documents.

Coordination of Assets: A will only controls assets that are titled in your name. You probably have other assets that are controlled by a contract, joint ownership or beneficiary designations; these include IRAs, 401(k)s, joint bank accounts, real estate and life insurance. A will does not control these assets. An experienced estate planning attorney will know how to coordinate these so that your assets are distributed the way you want.

Tax Planning: The federal estate tax exemption has been a moving target in recent years. Also, many states have their own death or inheritance tax, often at much lower exemptions than the federal tax.

Careful professional planning is a must in order to avoid paying too much federal or state tax.

Same Sex and Other "Living Together" Relationships: Because laws are frequently changing and vary greatly from state to state, it is vital to have updated advice from a competent professional. I have counseled couples who have lived together for 30 years or more. They intend to leave their property to each other, but without proper planning, many rights may be limited for unmarried cohabitants.

Complexity and Cost: Most people think their estate planning will be simple. The reality is, most people discover they need some personalized planning…and you may not know that without the guidance and counseling of an experienced attorney. It is far better to spend a little money and effort now to make sure your plan is created correctly than to try to save a few dollars and have things turn out badly later. You will not be around then to straighten things out.

Here are some things you can do to help keep costs down:

Become an educated consumer. The more you learn and understand about estate planning, the less time an attorney will need to spend educating you about the process.

Prepare a list of assets and liabilities and gather relevant documents (deeds, titles, beneficiary designations, etc.).

Consider beneficiaries and any special needs they may have.

Shop around a bit. Ask friends and acquaintances for referrals. If costs are a concern, let the attorney know up front that you are concerned about costs;

the attorney may be willing to work with you to keep them as low as possible.

Consider what you think you want, but be open to the attorney's suggestions.

# 29

# PREVENTING THE FIGHTS AFTER YOU'RE GONE

The single most important way to prevent your loved-ones from arguing after you are gone or when you are incapacitated is to be very clear about your wishes in legally binding, written documents.

Families fight for a number of reasons. Sometimes, arguments ensue simply because the people who love you have different opinions on how to best care for you or carry out your wishes. If this is the reason your family fights, it is your fault for leaving unclear directions.

Other times, family fights occur because of greed. I have noticed over the last decade a significant increase in the number of cases where the spouse winds up sued by the dead person's children (in other words, the wife or husband is sued by the step-kids). If you are a blended family, you have a very strong incentive to make your wishes clear to your spouse and to your children. Relying on the probate court to sort out your wishes is lunacy. I have even seen cases where the newly married couple took the time to prepare a prenuptial agreement as well as estate planning documents, but did not keep either updated. Changes to beneficiaries on retirement plans and life insurance policies as they went through the years together seemed "normal" and "common sense" to the couple, but not to the kids, who were given a copy of the prenuptial agreement by a well-meaning, newly remarried parent decades prior to the parent's death. If you create documents and then share them with your children, you also need to make sure you share your updated plans with your children. They often do not care as much for your new partner as you might.

Below are the top estate planning failures that give families the fuel to fight in court:

**Unclear Documents.** Most of the documents that are involved in will contests or other litigation were drafted by people without legal advice from a licensed and competent attorney. Please note that paralegals have not gone to law school, cannot give legal advice, and usually do not have any kind of malpractice insurance to protect you if they make a mistake.

**Outdated Documents.** Your life circumstances will likely change after you create your estate plan. If your documents are not updated to reflect the changes in your family and financial situation, you can be certain that people will argue about your estate when you are gone or how to care for you if you are incapacitated. One of the most commons "fights" in this situation is between natural children and your new spouse. If you took the time to create a prenuptial agreement, but later ignored it, you need to take the time to formally dissolve the prenuptial agreement, or your children may try to enforce it after you are gone when you no longer want it enforced. If you create conflicting documents, your family will argue and likely spend much of the estate on attorneys.

**The Problem Child.** If you have a child who is estranged, you should create a trust plan, not a will plan. Why? Because your disinherited child will be "invited" by the court system to contest the will. If you use a trust, on the other hand, and you do not leave the problem child anything – not even $1.00 – then that child is not a beneficiary of the trust and has no right to a copy of the trust in most states. Most ethical attorneys will be very reluctant to pursue a lawsuit when they cannot see a copy of the trust your child might claim exists ahead of time.

**Competency Issues.** Another reason to use an attorney when preparing your documents is that the lawyer, after your incapacity or death, can become your best witness. It is much harder for disgruntled heirs to turn your plan upside down when a lawyer will testify that they asked you many questions about your assets and your family, and that they are certain you understood the consequences of the legal documents.

Competent estate planning attorneys will also make sure they meet with you alone, without any children in the room, so they can document that your decisions were not influenced by a manipulative child or any other person.

In the above ways, your estate planning attorney is not only your guide and counselor with years of experience to help you make your decisions, but your attorney can also be your best witness if someone tries to upset your careful planning.

Made in the USA
Middletown, DE
04 July 2023